THE STROKER

By

Danzie Stewart

THE STROKER

By

Danzie Stewart

First Edition 2015
Danzie Stewart
Birmingham, UK
Copyright © 2015 Danzie Stewart
Published by Danzie Stewart, Birmingham, UK
ISBN 978-1-905028-10-8

Acknowledgements

I would like to acknowledge the help of my former partner Cascia Davis, my family, Dr. Mel Thompson, my niece Novlette Reece, Alvin Henry and Occupational Therapy, for their invaluable help, support and encouragement with this book.

DEDICATION

To Mum and Dad

WITH LOVE

Contents

Foreword

Stroke is the brain equivalent of a heart attack. There are approximately 152,000 strokes a year in the UK, resulting in 49,000 deaths.[1]

At any given time there are over 900,000 people living with disabilities as a result of a stroke.

According to the stroke association statistics October 2006, the incidence of stroke is higher in African Caribbean people who are twice as likely to have strokes compared with Caucasian people. As an African Caribbean person, I believe this is due to a combination of issues foremost of which are: stress, diet and lifestyle.

Although the incidence of stroke increases with age, anyone can have a stroke. Strokes are known to have occurred in babies.

I hope that this account of my experience, having had three strokes, which have changed my life, relationships and world view, will throw some light on some of the un-chartered areas of that journey.

---

1   Townsend, N. *et al* (2012) Coronary Heart Disease Statistics, British Heart Foundation, 20, 57

THE EVENT

At 2.00am, on the second Sunday in April that year, my life fell apart and changed forever; but little did I know it then, or could even have guessed. For a couple of weeks previously, I had been experiencing some headiness and the odd period of dizziness. This was a familiar, but thankfully an infrequent visitor.

This particular night, I had been to the birthday party of a friend who lived next door on the estate. The party was a cosy affair, attended by another neighbour and his wife. I had been to such parties before, and we usually ended up talking about old times.

True to form, we soon fell into well-trodden roles. Ken another friend of the host, led off the session and held sway with descriptions of by gone days, when Britain was the work shop of the world. In those days you could walk from one factory to many others in the industrial part of the city, and be offered two or three jobs in an afternoon.

The host who, at mid eighty, was the eldest member of the group, who spoke so quietly that you had to listen hard to hear him, played his role of respected elder. We were all very fond of him and dead quiet would reign when he spoke. This encouraged his discourse; he would keep the conversation flowing with juicy bits of reminiscences, some of which were quite irreverent. Ken's wife and I were the usual participants, chipping in when we got a chance to. This was right up our street because we were usually too tired to do much else.

The visitation of my malady at the party led me to make a decision to leave. This time the dizziness felt somehow different and a little bit scary. I was somewhat unhappy about having to leave early, but I explained to the host that I was not feeling one hundred per cent, and he understood. We were all coping with regular ups and downs in relation to our health, and we were very supportive towards each other, at that end of the estate.

I went straight home, and after fumbling with the front door key for some time, I had forgotten to replace the blown porch light, I managed to get the key into the slot. I then had my customary wash and went straight to bed.

I must have slept a little because when I next looked at the clock it was almost 2.00am. I remembered I was teaching the following day and reached for the book I was reading in preparation. I put it down when my vision became blurred, assuming that my eyes had simply got tired. I felt disorientated, and experienced the not unfamiliar sensation of floating in the bed; simultaneously the ceiling seemed to swirl, and the whole room to kaleidoscope, like a scene from Vertigo, an old Alfred Hitchcock movie.

That's how it felt sometimes when I was about to have a major angina attack. Normally, a frantic search for the glycerine pump, a puff or two, a dash for water, and a prayerful plea for more time, would settle the crisis down. But this time I did not get a chance to put those things into action. It was only when I rolled over; in an attempt to get out of bed and fell onto the wooden floor, with a resounding thud, that I began to understand the enormity of what had happened to me.

I HAD BEEN HIT BY A STROKE.

For a few moments I froze in disbelief and panic. Suddenly, the public health notice I had seen on TV, flashed in front of what was left of my mind. It had said, when stroke strikes, act fast. The faster you act the more of the person you save. Being alone in the house, I was in deep trouble. I needed to act, and to get help fast. I made several unsuccessful attempts to stand and finally decided to crawl the few yards to the living room, which I used as my study and where the telephone was kept. Still on the floor, I managed to drag the telephone off the old pine table, which served as my desk.

But who would I call? In ordinary circumstances I would have no hesitation identifying the need for an ambulance in response to a serious medical crisis. However, on this occasion it never occurred to me. It was as if a part of my mind could not accept what had happened to me, without some form of independent confirmation. My family would be overwhelmed with shock, fear, and concern. They were likely to panic, and it would take them some time to decide what to do.

Having blocked out calling an ambulance, and deciding that I could not contact my family at that stage, I still had to make a decision as to who else I could contact. My partner, who I usually saw at least every fortnight, lived too far away to be a realistic proposition. She lived in London, which was over a hundred miles from me. Even if I could wake her up, because of the distance she could not be of any direct help, although she would want to.

I decided I would ring my good friend Ula who was a health visitor, had spent most of her life in the medical profession, and had held a wide range of specialist and managerial nursing experience. She was used to keeping a calm head in a situation of crisis. She would know what to do immediately. I had met Ula when, as a young social worker, I had moved back to Birmingham, from Yorkshire, to be with my ill father, who had cancer of the blood, melanoma, from which he eventually died.

Up to the time of his fatal illness he was a fit man who hardly went down with anything, not even flu. So the family had great difficulty in coming to terms with his death, at the comparatively early age of sixty five. But his death would have been in any case, experienced as a great loss by many people because he was well

16

loved by his family and church. He was the pastor of the church and was a very charismatic man and a dynamic preacher. He was loved and admired not only by his congregation but by many others in his local community.

There was a widely held rumour that his illness was caused by drinking dirty water on his last missionary trip to Africa. It was unlikely but it provided a partial outlet for those who needed something or somebody to blame, in order to deal with their heavy grief.

I had seen Ula at a joint meeting between Health and Social Services, which was held in a local church hall that is still being hired out for meetings, up to the present day. That was in the days before I finally learned, that a lot of social work time was taken up by meetings, and that I needed to be very decisive about which ones I attended.

Her narrow face reminded me of a picture of Nefertitti, an ancient Queen of Egypt and who was reputed to be the mother of Tutankhamen. The golden death mask of this young god prince is probably the most familiar representation of Egyptian art. At that time, I was going through my Black consciousness, African self-discovery phase, which for some Black people, it seems to me, never appear to grow out of, and continue to idolised all things African.

I was amazed at how slender Ula was. She was by far

the slimmest woman in the hall, although I did not take a close, fine, detailed look at her, for fear of causing embarrassment. I was a bit attracted to Ula but had never thought of having a man-woman relationship with her. She was a devout Seventh Day Adventist, of the fundamentalist order. Their strict codes of behaviour set them apart in everyday life.

We both worked in the same locality but I never saw her for weeks afterwards. Then one afternoon I was returning home from my final visit of the day, in my cherished, metallic blue, Toyota Celica, which was quite rare at the time, when I spotted her. She was sloping along the pavement on a familiar road, which I had travelled since childhood.

I drove the car along-side her and reached over and opened the passenger door. In my nervousness I blurted, "Get in." Incredibly, she did and I gave her a lift home. I never found out why she accepted my rather unconventional approach, and why she rode with me that day. But we have been good friends ever since; for over thirty years.

It's just as well, because for a long time after my stroke, my vision was impaired, making it impossible for me to read. During that period, I needed help with my correspondence. She was one of the only two people, I would trust with my business; the only other person I trusted with my business was my partner who could not be with me every week.

18

However, Ula was looking after her elderly mother who had reached the prominent age of 94, as far as she knew. In reality she might have been much older. But surely Ula would not mind my ringing so late in this particular situation. It's not every day that something like this happened. Ula liked to go to bed early and was a good sleeper. I knew that she usually liked to be in bed by 9.00pm. Nonetheless, I decided she was the right person to ring.

Crawling the few yards along the floor from the bedroom to my office, I reached for the phone which was kept on the old pine table which acted as my desk. I turned it towards me. When I attempted to grasp it, I got my second shock. My hands could not grasp the telephone, but it did not stop there. There was more and it got worse. My eyes could not make out the numerals.

Momentary panic set in, I would have had to get help without the telephone. Then it dawned on me; it would have to be the neighbours. I would have needed to reach them somehow. I would have to get to them by crawling but it was two o'clock in the morning. Surely, no one would be awake at that time. Nevertheless, I was desperate. I had to try.

Luckily I had left the key in the latch, and whilst lying on the floor, I managed to reach up with my left hand which was only partly affected by paralysis, and pushed open the front door. It was a chrome grey half-moon night, which was clear enough for nocturnal activity yet left enough shadows for hiding if the need arose. On the open drive it gave no cover for my unusual and humiliating style of traverse.

As I set off down my drive I was struck by unexpected pain from a surface I thought was negotiable because it looked smooth. It was not. I found out the hard way when the reality imprinted itself in my mind, as each pebble and indentation roughly introduced itself to me. In the images I previous had of concrete surfaces, they had always been smooth. This experience at close proximity was a surprise as I felt the many irregularities and extrusions of all shapes and sizes.

Dragging myself along I had started to make my way down the drive, to my neighbour on the left, Mr White, when I realised that I could not endure much more pain. I was not going to make it that way. The neighbour to the left, whose party I had attended earlier, would be rather too far. It would have involved going about twelve yards to the bottom of my drive, along the road to the left for almost as many yards, circumventing the dividing fence, then up his drive to the front door.

My neighbours to the right Ken, was a better prospect. My home was separated from theirs by only the few yards of narrow tarmac driveway giving access to his garage which was adjoining mine. Both garages with their flat roofs looked like little prefabricated houses. All I would have to do, was to make my way directly across to the right to get to their front door. I slowly and painfully made my way across, propelling myself with my least affected arm and legs. In this way exerting myself to the limit, I managed to reach my neighbour, Ken's house. I clawed and pushed myself up Ken's front door, to achieve a vertical position, and knocked.

I gave it all I had and knocked as hard as I could, which was probably not very hard. Panic set in and I started to seriously doubt the wisdom of my decision. Surely they would not be up at that time of night. A few moments passed. I was about to go and try to think of something else, when I decided to try just one more time - this time for luck. I was surprised when Alison opened the door and leaned her head out. Close behind her was Ken. They took one look at me and must have realized I was ill. One of them immediately threw a blanket over my shoulders.

In my preoccupation with getting help I had become oblivious to the weather and how chilly it was outside. Ken's warm blanket was a welcomed contrast and assurance of safety. Ken half carried and supported me to a chair in the kitchen. He proceeded to give me water to drink, cupping his hand underneath and bearing the weight of the glass himself. He and his wife then made gentle reassuring small talk. I followed only fragments of their conversation, whilst I tried to hold my fluctuating consciousness together.

At one point I tried to explain what had happened, but found that normal speech had disappeared. I managed to gurgle sufficiently coherently, what they already knew, that I had a stroke and needed an ambulance. They must have dialled it without my knowing because a few seconds later one arrived. The paramedics came into the kitchen and made enquiries in such muted and respectful voices, it would easily have been possible to think that I was close to my final journey. This may not have been far from the truth, for Ken told me afterwards, that when he saw me on that occasion, I looked like a dead man.

The paramedics were two Caucasian men, both were above average height but one was significantly taller than the other. The shorter one was a little plump and heading for fat which possibly made him look shorter than he really was. I suddenly became unusually conscious of their smell. Both smelt fresh and clean with a hint of something else. It was like the delicate aroma of Chinese chicken. If it was an ethnic attribute, I speculated that other groups must have their own and I thought, black people must have a smell as well.

But if there was such a thing as ethnic smell, being African Caribbean, I had lost the sense of my own ethnic smell through constant exposure. In the same way that I lost the smell of Cadbury's chocolate, after a week of attending college near the factory where they make the stuff. I have lost the awareness of my own smell, and African Caribbean's are very good at

22

covering our own smell. It was an essential part of personal grooming and self-presentation. This also embraced hair and skin care, and appropriate dress.

From early childhood we are taught to avoid abrasive admonitions such as, 'your skin looks white like chalk', or it 'looks like leather', and 'your hand feel like lizard'. Similarly when your hair appeared to need attention, persons may state mockingly, that 'it was dry like chips', or that it was 'coarse like crocus bag' (a crocus bag made from rough fibres) and 'thick like horse's hair'.

This would usually be followed by detailed questioning as to whether and when you had washed yourself in carbolic or scented soap, and applied pomade to your hair. For some reason this was always of the American variety. You would become aware of it as soon as a pomaded person walked into the room. This would be vigorously applied with massage movement, towards the centre and outside of the scalp alternatively.

Your mother, female relatives, or close friend, would then take your hands in hers, and liberally apply a dollop of moisturising lotion which we called cold cream, to your face and hands. A favourite horn comb would be drawn repeatedly through your hair, regardless of the howls caused by its encounter with your tangled tuffs and snags.

A detailed finger inspection would then take place.

The magic of the moment would be followed by a long lingering look, and the ceremony of the occasion would be ended, by a slight squeeze of the hand, or a couple of playful slaps, just below the buttocks. You would pull your mouth close, and pout your lips, in a mock show of manly nonchalant, to disguise the fact that, you secretly enjoyed it.

Neither your family nor friends were aware of the origin of this particular type of grooming. Nor did they know of its cultural links with African displacement to the Caribbean, the Diaspora and slavery. A central feature of slavery was that Africans were forced through a process of re-socialization to condition them to believe that all things white were good and was to be esteemed. While all things Black were bad and were to be shunned or 'whitified'.

An African was not allowed to be regarded as acceptable until he had been through this process. In this way Kunta Kente, in Alex Haley's "Roots", was not acceptable until he adopted his European name. As the African slave was discouraged from maintaining his culture, his language and religion, and so, he was encouraged to take on the culture of the slave master. The process was accompanied by severe punishment for descent and rewarded according to compliance.

Out of this process developed a powerful, unexpected, psychological mechanism which proved useful to the slave master. Many slaves not only came to love their

24

oppressors, but actively wanted to look like him and to take on his culture and values. Hence, hair and skin care also became a means of looking less African, more like the master and more acceptable to Europeans.

Over a period of time, this developed into a full scale preoccupation with personal presentation, which embraced not only looking good, but also smelling the best you could afford. The preoccupation has been passed down from one generation to the next. Although the origins and meaning has been mostly lost, the practice still exists among Black people of the Diaspora.

Speculating on the distinct smell of the two white paramedics, I decided that only some white people smelt that way, since most of the white people I had known did not. If that was the case it was likely that some Black people had a distinctive smell as well. How then would I explain my experience with the two white physios. It's a longstanding held belief among Black people of the Diaspora, that white people smell different. This I have heard said, as a child, by some of my family and friends.

It was difficult to separate serious assertions from the type of group stereotyping which has been going on between black and white people for generations. Some people are so convinced of the rightness of this view that they are prepared to go on TV to assert them; as happened on the Oprah Winfrey show a few years ago.

Having had a personal experience which appeared to support this, it is understandable that you can't help wondering whether there is something there.

Perhaps distinctive types of smell were confined to pure blooded people; but no such group exists. Medical conditions such as sickle cell anaemia and thalassemia, supposed to be only in Africans, African-Caribbeans and Asians, have been found in northern Europeans. Furthermore, the University of California, have traced the origins to modern man by his DNA, and have found that he originated in North Africa. All the respected scientific evidence supports this.

We share a common gene pool which has been mixed and remixed by different waves of migration commencing with the first which spread humans from our birthplace. We all originated in Africa and within all of us regardless of ethnicity are the genetic imprint of our first African mother.

While I was in hospital recovering from my recent stroke, out of sheer boredom I made up a game of 'I can guess who you are from your smell'. People were always going and coming from the ward; most were medical staff and tended to follow predictable timetables according to their shifts. In this game I would close my eyes and see if I could recognize the individuals who came on to the ward, by their smell. I had some success in this game because most people wore distinctive smelling fragrances, perfumes and deodorant, which were easy to recognise.

I also had some notable failures as well. They came when there were people who did not appear to have a smell which was detectable from where I was and where several people wore the same thing. A particular deodorant was so common among some members of the nursing staff, I got to wondering whether it was NHS general issue. No ethnic pattern was detectable and it was a Caribbean woman that stood out the most; it was she who smelt noticeably the strongest, it was unmistakable. I was aware of her whenever she entered the ward. I am sure her colleagues were aware of it too but, perhaps out of respect, chose not to react.

Historically white people, particularly those directly involved in the enslavement of Black people, have held negative beliefs about them. The modern day version, in regards to smell, was clearly expressed when Black people from the Caribbean and later the wider commonwealth, started to come here in large numbers, in the 1950s.

According to this view, Black people stank of the oil they used on their hair and skin. Now the irony is that moisturising the hair and skin have become so much a part of popular culture, you can hardly watch television for a quarter of an hour without seeing some advert extolling the virtues of some hair oil or skin lotion. These suggest, persuasively, that you would be incomplete without whatever brand is being proffered. Of this only I feel sure, all unadorned flesh smells, if you get close enough to detect it, individuals smell differently and some stronger than others. Some people are more aware of it than others, and are more successful at disguising it.

Everyone wants to smell good and of those who don't, few were soap shy. For the overwhelming majority of people who do not smell good, physical, social or environmental circumstances beyond their control, is to blame. My experience following my stroke bears witness to this. About six months after my stroke, I started to notice that people around me were sniffing in my direction and subtly, steer away from me; including family and friends. Then it suddenly hit me. It was me they were sniffing at and that I smelt; it was a smell of urine.

I was horrified and experienced a mixture of strong feelings. I was overwhelmed with shame and felt excluded from the ranks of whole people. But I also experienced anger at being treated like a leper, even by members of my own family. How easy it was to fall into the role of purer than thou, and to forget the feelings of others, however near or dear.

When I checked myself, I noticed from damp underpants that I was leaking. Not just the trickle that many men find running down their trousers, often resulting in a cold shock, after going to the loo; but more. I was so alarmed that it kept me preoccupied for weeks trying different things, in a hunt for a cure, some of which were downright risky. Until a solution was found I went through social hell and suffered agonies.

I was so desperate that I shared it with my sympathetic occupational therapist. I was amazed when she told me, to my great relief, that it was a common occurrence among people of my age, people who had a stroke and particularly among women. She also shared that women had good days and bad. They had a simple way of dealing with it, when they were having a bad day they wore scented panty liners. They could be obtained economically, from all major supermarkets.

Armed with this information I decided to venture forth and find out what the NHS could offer to tide me over until a permanent solution was sought. The large pads I ended up with, curtsy of the local health visitor, were absorbent enough, but did little to mask the smell. So I fell back on the information from occupational health, and got my women friends and sisters to buy me scented liners.

Whatever the truth regarding bodily smells, I have discovered that since my stroke I am more aware of them. It's not as if I can smell more acutely, like Jack Nicholson, in the film, 'Wolfe.' But when your other senses are diminished, you tend to make better use of what you have left.

I was surprised that I had ventured into racial theorising which was against my personal values and which I felt well guarded against. I had spent many years teaching race equality to a large spectrum of people, professional and unqualified. Perhaps the stroke either brought to the surface aspects of me which had previously been buried, or a change in my personality had occurred.

After a little while the ambulance men gently lifted me onto a metal framed wheel chair: that they re-organised as a stretcher once we were outside. This was not too dissimilar from the trolley you see at funerals, bringing the body into church. I was moved from the stretcher to a slightly wider and much more substantial platform, once inside the vehicle. I can imagine the sound of sirens from the ambulance and the blurred shapes of houses, lamp posts and a few nocturnal strays flashing by as we dashed through the night. But I was unaware of it, for the next thing I knew was that we had arrived at the hospital.

Thankfully they did not cannulise me as other paramedics had done on previous emergencies. I have always found this to be a painful procedure, having inherited the family trait, deep vein which were difficult to find. Usually it required several attempts at finding them and each attempt involved puncturing the skin. It did not take a long time before you began to feel like an abused pin cushion, which was accompanied by serious pain.

So I was glad they did not try to fit a cannula. But they did fix a transparent plastic mask over the top of my face, and gave me oxygen. With my stroke warped speech and oxygen mask, they did not stand much chance of getting much coherent speech out of me. They must have got the information they needed from Alison and Ken, for I was able to nod confirmation to the questions they asked, and which was really a means of calming me.

THE RECEPTION

I do not recall much about the dizzy journey. I kept moving in and out of consciousness as the paramedics rushed to see how much of me they could save. If I was just an assignment in a busy schedule, which I most likely was, they did not show it. Even if it was just another day at the office, they showed great care and humanity. I remembered being carried from the mobile stretcher to a bed, located in a cubicle in the emergency reception area. The cubicle had one end open; this was the end facing me. So I had a full view of much of my immediate surroundings.

I am not sure whether Ken and Alison had driven ahead or whether they had followed the ambulance, but when I got to the A & E they appeared. I was then taken through A & E to the emergency waiting area and to a cubicle. After a few minutes in the cubicle I was seen by a young nurse. Perhaps out of youthful enthuse she attempted an interview in a manner which felt like an interrogation. Needless to say it ended in a rather one sided interaction with her reading my personal details, presumably which came from my files, for this was my local hospital, and my croaking and nodding in response. When she left Ken and Alison came in.

Alison and Ken again made light conversation of the sort they would do, if you had gone around to their home for a mid-week drink or cup of tea. They stayed until other people arrived. After them Ulna and then my sisters were next on the scene. Alice and Ken were really great; it was so reassuring to share such a frightening part of my journey, with people I knew. To have them there was so helpful while I was still in a state of shock and trying to find my balance, after what had happened to me.

I appeared to be facing the office. And saw nurses moving about, some hastily, but always in a controlled manner. I was surprised by the large number of male nursing staff, many of them by their mannerisms and speech, appeared gay. This left me thinking how far behind the times I was, and how much social change had happened. How did this leave women patients feeling? In law women still had a choice in relation to personal care as to whether they wanted to receive a service from a woman or man.

They could refuse to have personal care from a man. Not many women appeared to exercise this choice. Paradoxically there was evidence to suggest that large numbers of women did not mind and some actually preferred to be cared for by a man. My nurse was female. She first examined my oxygen mask then disappeared and then came back with a callunar. This appeared smaller than usual and it did not hurt too much whilst it was being inserted, or afterwards. In my previous experience with cannulas, any major movement would give you jip.

I imagined that there were specific small ones for people who were obviously genuine cases, and there was an unequivocal desire to cause the least distress. But patients, whose sincerity was questionable, were not treated so sensitively.

The nurse who attended me and who I thought of as 'mine' although I saw her going to other cubicles, was as sweet as a Caribbean damsel with a saintly smile and up curved lips. It was the sort of beauty you wanted to hold onto, not just savour as a last reminder of what was good in this world. That was when I had my first suspicion that I was going to live. I was going to come through and somehow survive.

She attempted to take some brief details about my medical background leading up to the stroke, and which I had previously been through already. I tried to assist her as much as I could, with my limited communication capacity, despite a gathering annoyance as to how many times I would have to repeat the same information and tell the same story. She then told me that the doctor would see me soon.

She then asked me and my visitors, if we wanted some tea. My two sisters and I had one. Ulna remained behind but did not have a drink. I wondered whether the nurse was following normal practice or if this was simply a case of individual kindness. If it was the latter, given the cut backs, she was likely to get into trouble at some stage. With the cut backs had come a tightening of the rules. Nurses were only supposed to give NHS refreshments to patients.

Finally the doctor arrived. He seemed more true to a traditional expectation of role, but then my exposure to such a kaleidoscope of gender, sexual and ethnic mix, was forcing me to re-examine my image of the norm within the service. The doctor asked for a more detailed account of what had happened to me, from my evening crisis, what had followed, up to the point when I arrived at the A & E. He also enquired about how my experience had affected me.

Initially he asked to speak to me alone and everyone else left the cubicle. However when the going soon became rough, he asked my sisters to join us. They were more able to tell the story, based on what they had heard from Alison and Ken. Some were based on my own gurgles. They also seemed able to interpret them.

Normally I would have been very annoyed that I had to give much of the same information, in quick succession, to several people working in the same department. I actually started to become so, but I was so mentally fazed that it did not seem to matter. Time passed and a couple of hours went by without event. I was beginning to feel abandoned, when a porter and nurse appeared. Without much ado they pushed my narrow bed out of the cubicle and into the reception area.

I felt a momentary drop in temperature, as I was pulled and pushed along narrow corridors with magnolia painted walls. These were interspersed, at regular intervals, by double doors leading into wards. After travelling along a long corridor we came to the reception ward. I did not know it at the time, but it was to be my new home for a while.

The ward was a long oblong sleeve with beds arranged on both sides and a narrow walk way, sufficiently wide for the passage of hospital beds, medical equipment and meal trolleys, all of which were on wheels. My bed was located on the left hand side, third from the end. It was surrounded by warm drapes which gave my position a cosy private comforting feel. A psychotherapist might say it gave an illusion of a womb experience. And at that time it was something like that I needed; to be comforted! Except for nights, of which I was blissfully unaware, I spent the first two days, in a state of semi-consciousness.

Sri Lankan Woman

Despite my sometimes, partial grip on consciousness, I was aware that the ward was staffed mostly by Asians, the majority of whom were Orientals. At first I thought it unusual but I was not surprised. They had comprised the great majority of the staff at my late cousin's nursing home, and had been his carers before he died horribly from emphysema. He had been struggling for each breath, after three years on an oxygen machine.

In his better days, most of his immediate family, including his eight children and numerous nephews and nieces, indulged his boasts about continuous chain smoking and boozing, from dawn till dusk. But with the exception of two of his daughters, they hardly visited him in his later years of suffering, although they nearly all attended his funeral. It was I and two of his daughters who took close interest in him. One daughter lived in the same town as me, which was not too far away from him. We used to visit together until she bought her own car. The other lived in the same town as he did and it was convenient for her to visit him.

She stayed close when he was moved from his warden supported flat to a nursing home and later, during his spells in hospital. I am not sure whether her motives were purely daughterly though. For within a few days following his death, while everyone was still reeling with grief, she went to his flat and behind everyone's back, she cleaned out all his possessions.

In good African and Caribbean tradition, his relatives in this country all turned up for his funeral. This was despite their not having seen him in years or during his illness when he needed them most. I was so angered by this hypocrisy, that I could not help mentioning how they had treated him and had let him down. My speech was contrary to funeral tradition of inflating the deceased and giving comfort to the bereaved. My feelings were so strong that I did not care.

The care I received from the Asian staff was excellent. They were not only very diligent and gentle; they were tireless in attending to my needs. There was one particular Asian nurse who stayed in my mind. She was an Oriental type, with a narrow face and was very pretty. It was she who was assigned to me. She took an almost personal devotion to my care. So I was only partly embarrassed, and not my customary, very uncomfortable self, when on several occasions I had to call for a bed pan. But only for a wee, not for a number two!

I think she sensed that I liked her; for we got into conversation and she eventually told me she was from Sri Lanka. I had never met anyone from there, before.

But I left the ward before I could ask her about how she came to be here. She did give me her name and address written on a pale blue, personal card. The state of my mind and emotions were such that I did not take her gesture seriously. She left the ward before me and like a holiday friendship, once she had left thoughts of her soon disappeared. But she was important for my emotional and psychic revival. Not only was I going to survive, I was still going to be able to be a man.

INITIATION

At about mid-day on my third day, I found myself being lifted from my bed to a slightly narrower mobile affair. However, it was when it appeared that I was being moved out of the ward and along intolerably long corridors, that I suspected something that significant was afoot. I was being moved unexpectedly to another ward. This was happening without any preparation or fore warning. No one had mentioned anything about it to me.

The orderlies were sure-footed and clear about where we were going. But the fact that I had received no inkling and that I was to be moved left me in a state of bemusement if not confusion. My fragile equanimity was rippled, but I had experienced nothing to suggest that I was not going to be all right. Well, that certainty was the case, before I experienced the late night staff, on my new ward. My journey terminated with my being wheeled around, from forward facing to backwards, into a ward. I was entered through double doors, with twin rectangular, fire resistant, translucent glass, panels.

The ward was long and rectangular, divided by a broad concourse. At the entrance end, on the left hand side as you entered the ward, there was a kitchen, toilets and shower rooms. Further down the ward the space was divided into staff facilities and storage areas. To the right, opposite the kitchen and bathrooms, was the day room and physio unit. Below the unit, the area was partitioned into three dormitories. These were really mini wards. Each dormitory had two rows of six beds, one on either side of a passage, a bit narrower than the central concourse.

The ward was staffed by a more traditional compliment of health care workers. This was a mixture of British people, a substantial proportion of people of Irish extraction, several female Caribbean nurses, and one Oriental, female nurse. Half the doctors were Asian and there were a couple of Africans. Had Enoch Powell lived, he would have had a fit to discover, the role the people he had played a leading part in recruiting from the commonwealth, would come to hold. These were the people he later thought, would be responsible for creating rivers of blood, in this country, and who have come to share, a crucial part of the responsibility, for maintaining the nation's health.

My bed in the new ward was on the right side of the second dormitory, at the beginning of the row. I was opposite the nurse's station. Beds were situated adjacent to me and further up the row behind me. With the staff station in front of me, I was surrounded on all sides. Being a creature of privacy I felt uncomfortably exposed. Initially I was a little put out that I had been

44

placed in this position. But I reasoned that, as a new-be on the ward, I was too uncertain of the ward norms or my status in the pecking order, to push the boat out. I needed to get settled and get to know the 'runnings' before I could make any demands.

And so, I let my two feeble attempts at achieving greater privacy, by half drawing the surrounding screen, be thwarted by two unknown nurses. As soon as they saw the screen, out of what they considered to be the right position, they drew them back, and marched off before I could say anything.

The dormitories were open plan and from my advantageous position opposite the work station, I had a good view of what went on at that part of the ward. The work station was occupied by the ward sister, most of the time when she was on duty. The exceptions were, when she was called away or, vacated it for a desk at the other end of the ward, in order to use the computer there. The vacant workstation gave someone else a chance for a break away from ordinary duties. This they invariably used to make telephone calls; I suspected, mostly of a personal nature, at the expense of the N.H.S. It also gave me an unintended opportunity to play at character assessment. Most staff appeared delighted with this temporary oasis.

Some staff would try to cover their pleasure, but not with complete success, as they occupied the favoured position with glee. Others would puff themselves up and assume an extra whiff of self-importance. The only people who appeared unchanged were a taciturn female English nurse, and a Chinese looking male nurse. They contrasted noticeably with the majority of staff, who showed their satisfaction, in some subtle, almost indefinable, way.

The prolonged use of the ward telephone by staff could sometimes be a bit frustrating, as it barred patients, including myself, from using it. This was not usually a problem for staff, as they had mobiles. Patients never had the courage to complain. They exercised patience, or simply suffered in silence. Eventually some decided to surreptitiously sneak in their own mobiles. I eventually asked one of my sisters to bring in mine. I was met with a bemused look and a half smile, as I plugged the charger, into a hospital socket.

As I came onto the ward, a health care worker in a manila, grey striped, uniform, looked over my bedding, and made final adjustments. I could not quite work out whether this was to ensure my comfort or to maintain ward standards of decorum. Apart from that, no one took any interest in me, or thought to ask me whether I had eaten, or to offer me anything. I was a freshman on the ward and too much of a newcomer to say anything to staff. I suppose I thought someone would eventually notice me. That's what I would have liked. But no one did; certainly not where my need for food was concerned.

I did not want to appear demanding, or to make waves. I wanted to suss things out slowly. And it was as well that I did. As no one enquired whether I had eaten I watched lunch and then dinner go by. I didn't mind too much, about the missed meals. I am naturally a light eater; whose attitude to food, my dad once described as like, a student stomach.

I also knew I wouldn't starve because my partner and sisters had anticipated that I would experience, some less than satisfactory treatment in this area. So they had ensured that I was well stocked with lots of cartons of fruit juices and lemonade which I liked, fruits, packets of biscuits, and home cooked food. This I shared with my Asian neighbour who occupied the bed next to mine. He was a big man who got rather hungry and seemed to find the hospital meals insufficient, to the point where he was reduced to licking his plate, quite openly in public.

After witnessing that, I felt I had to intervene. I explained the situation to his relatives, in private, when they came to visit him, and suggested they bring him food from home. They did and the following day, his table was a washed with food. Many hours went by, no one gave me an explanation as to why I had been moved to this ward. No one enquired whether I had eaten or needed anything. No one spoke to me.

So I watched the meal times go, and watched other patients eat, whilst I tried to figure out what was going on. I concluded that there was nothing sinister going on. I had just been forgotten because I had not been assigned to any one in particular. I and my personal needs had been forgotten in the busy machinery of everyday hospital routine.

Things were shaping into a familiar symptom of a system under great stress. However I couldn't anticipate what was to follow, later that evening. Neither could any other patient, otherwise no one would allow themselves to be admitted to that ward; nor would anyone want to stay overnight at that hospital. I began to become aware of how, in the absence of vigilant and caring relatives, people could lose weight, become malnourished, or even starve, in hospital. They simply get overlooked, neglected and forgotten.

This process was enabled by staff shortages and by a deficient system for monitoring and ensuring, that all the patient needs were being addressed. This would inevitably cover the area of diet. This needs to be given the importance of medical needs and clear lines of responsibility established for it. A particular area which was important to monitor and manage is the procedure by which new patients are informed of how to order, and how the order by which patients received their meals, is decided. On this ward it was done by way of a linear list, the order of which remained static. When a new person joined, they were simply added to the bottom of it.

In order to be on the list, once they had found out about the procedure, a patient had to either personally complete a request form or have it done on their behalf. This was normally done by a nurse, on the day before the meal was required. It usually took new patients some time to become familiar with this system, and they would miss meals until they did; or until they happened to be noticed by a member of the nursing staff, who would order it for them. They could never be guaranteed to be available when needed, or to remember that task. They were usually very busy.

Furthermore, once a patient got on the list, the waiting time for each meal was determined by their numerical ranking. I was once shown the list, after I had missed supper, for the second time, and was brought to their attention by my very assertive niece. She had demanded to see the list, to ensure that I was on it.

I was surprised to see that the list was some twenty patients long. I was second from the last, and it normally took over two hours to get to me. That was a long time to wait when you are hungry. It also appeared that the further down the list you were the greater the likelihood that you would be missed. This was a similar experience for other patients too. On several occasions I ended up sharing food with them, from the supply brought in by my family and friends.

Eventually I had to share my food secretly or when I was asked, because I overheard a comment one of the nurses made, about my generosity. It led me to believe, if I behaved like that too openly, they would interpret it, as evidence of mental illness. Being that far down the list, there was always the possibility that by the time it was your turn, you would have experienced hunger. Most staff followed the list regimentally. I was trying not to stir up things, but neither was I going to be forgotten. This turned out to be a decision I would later regret.

The time was coming close to nine o'clock, the afternoon and early evening nurses began to drift off duty and I did not see any sign of my medication. I mentioned to a chiselled faced nurse who moved like a tom boy, and who was constantly straightening the bottom half of her uniform, as if to avoid the men on the ward noticing the tops of her legs, or to remind herself that she was a woman. I informed her that I did not receive my medication which was usually given at 8.00pm. A few minutes later, she disappeared off the ward, having forgotten me. The day staff were replaced by the late night crew; an all Caribbean and I suspected, all Jamaican team.

The prospect of being cared for by my own compatriots was initially comforting. It felt as if I was back home. So I did not feel any apprehension in asking for my cot sides to be lowered. They made me feel boxed in like a prisoner. I had tried unsuccessfully to do it myself. I could not reach the control lever from the bed and particularly with the bars raised. I noticed a Caribbean stout, nurse with a fawn coloured boxer face, and a curly perm, that was becoming slightly scraggly, on her greying head, giving her the appearance of a character from Michael Jackson's "Thriller". I asked her to lower my cot sides, as politely as I could and made sure I used the word please.

"Ku ya" she said, using a Jamaican expression of derision. She followed up by asking, "Who do you think you are? Don't you know those are to keep you from falling out of bed?" I replied that I knew, but that I did not like feeling imprisoned. She smiled in disbelief, that I had the gaul to make such a request and hold to it after her explanation. She froze momentarily, as if trying to decide how to react next, but did nothing.

She began to walk off, when I lost my resolve, I did not want to earn the name of a trouble maker, and reminded her that it was her duty to care for me. She then turned and asked me if I did not know what ward that was. Then she told me, that it was a going home ward, implying that I would have to start doing things for myself. I was forced to make a bargaining with her. She would grant my request but only if I agreed not to have a drink, gesturing at the tea trolley, she was helping with.

It was as if I had entered into "The Matrix," a computer generated reality. It could not be real. It must be some sort of aberration. Nurses don't behave that way. I tried to push the event to the back of my mind, but I sensed she needed to be given something. I could not see that I had any chips to bargain with. I was not an addicted tea soak. I did not need a hot drink, I rationalised. I could get by perfectly well on my cartons of drinks. I was being taught a lesson. For what reason, I did not know. That rankled, but little did I know, this was only the first chapter, of a painfully heavy book.

Mortal Danger

At about 10.00pm, not having had any sight of my medication, and which I had reported to the day and early evening staff, I became worried that it may have been forgotten. I had watched the late-night staff for about half hour as they appear to have finish off their initial tasks. Then two of them walked over to the staff station, the sister's desk.

I was unable to walk unaided yet, but I decided to see if I could make my way to the staff station, to inform the nurses of my apparently being overlooked. I did not want to run the risk of appearing a nuisance by calling a nurse over, using the orange string which hung down over the head of each bed. I manoeuvred myself out of bed, and by resting most of my right side on the patient's table, which luckily, was on the right side of my bed, I was able to push myself, using my goodish left leg, pushed my way to the sister's desk.

A fair skinned, Jamaican nurse seemed to be in charge. She looked like the type; Jamaicans usually refer to as, "red people from St Elizabeth". She was a middle aged woman, who was not very tall, but Caribbean big and becoming rather large. I shared, that it seemed as if I may have been overlooked, as I had not been given my medication. She did not move a muscle or bat an eye. There was no reply to me in any shape or form. She appeared totally unaware of me, although I stood less than a yard away, looking at and waiting for her, for more than a moment. If I could have reached out my hand, but for my paralysis, I could have touched her.

Her lack of response was weird and left me chilled, so I did not hang around for long. I did see her looking quizzically at me, in a sidelong glance, as I turned to head back. By then I was too uncomfortable to stop for a verbal inter-change. During my struggle back to bed, I saw two nurses with Jamaican accents, by the staff station. One was just above average height, athletic built, with well-defined features. She was wearing her hair in a short neat, curly perm.

The other nurse was taller and also well built, but in a more rounded manner. She was wearing a dark blue top, and black trouser. She had big hair, a well-tended curly perm, high cheekbones and a roman nose, with the exception of her eyes, she looked good. Her overall appearance would certainly not have disgraced a celebrity fighting woman from Roman times, an "Amazon". In contrast however, her eyes appeared fixed in a perpetual half smile, as if always on martial guard. And her lips seemed constantly frozen, in sneering self-satisfaction.

These two appeared to have a close relationship with the nurse who seemed to be the one in charge, presumably "the sister". One of them or sometimes both, were usually never far from her. They were joined by three other members of staff who also gathered around the nurse's station, as if pulled by invisible magnets. Then, to my amazement, they all walked off the ward, and disappeared; leaving the ward totally without staff, and unattended, for over forty minutes!

When they reappeared, two nurses stopped at the top section of the ward, and two accompanied the sister. The middle aged Amazon one went back to the nurse's station. They spent some time in conversation then started to do their rounds, beginning on my dormitory. The Amazon, in a blue top and black trousers, commenced at one end, accompanied by the one with the good physique, "the athlete". And the sister started at the other end, on the row of beds opposite me.

She made a great show of tending to the other patients, and of giving them their medication. By the time she came to me, it was well after 11.00pm. When she eventually came to me, she offered me my medication. But I ended up not taking them. As she handed me the cocktail of two tablets and two capsules, one of the capsules fell apart. Inside was a lime coloured powder, the likes of which I had not seen before. She hurriedly scooped up the powder and fragments of capsule which had fallen on the bed without any comment.

My first thought was that it must have been an accident. The pharmacy had messed up. It was just one of those things. I should not pay it any attention, or let it worry me in any way but it did not feel right. In my many days this had not happened before. Could this be a warning?

Too many worrying things had happened. I was not prepared to fully trust the late night staff any more. I was not going to put, I dread to think, possibly my life, at risk. Nor did I feel safe in putting my life into the sister's hands, at least not yet. I would wait and see. I was not prepared to rest on the basis of blind faith in the medical profession.

Over the years there have been reports of doctors and nurses who have either deliberately or through gross bad practice gone on to harm or even kill their patients. Surely there must have been concerns about their practice, before they went on to harm or murder their victims. Sadly, it is usually after the event and when the police become involved or when there is a public outcry, that these concerns are treated seriously.

The case of Doctor Harold Shipman, and more recently, Staffordshire Hospital, illustrates the point. Shipman killed around one hundred people, and at Staffordshire Hospital, it took over one thousand deaths before there was a serious enquiry. The unreasoned faith in the medical profession; which we are all conditioned to since childhood, rationalises away continuously, any contrary evidence or belief. It does not stop except, where rare providence intervenes, when your life, is at risk.

The Abuse

Later that night, the events of the day kept floating around my mind, like a moth that had lost its way in a closed room. There seemed to be no way I could understand what had taken place or why. I could not sleep. I tossed and turned. I tried every conceivable position, but was unable to find a comfortable one, in the narrow hospital bed. This had not been a problem for me previously. Nor had it appeared to be one for other patients; except possibly my Asian neighbour. He used to stay up all night, and often wandered, with the bed clothes wrapped around him, like a roman toga.

I later confirmed that the bed should not have been a problem. I was told by my consultant, who I came to trust, that it was an expensive bed. It had apparently cost over two thousand pounds to buy and was made for comfort. Although in ordinary circumstances the hospital bed was comfortable enough, it was not my bed. My bed at home had cost only a fraction of the price of the hospitals. But it had taken me three goes to find. It was a special orthopaedic bed that I had got on special offer at a closing down sale.

And I thought it was unique. It had a solid pine base, which I could hardly lift, and certainly could not carry, was 1000 pocket sprung, and had an orthopaedic centre area in the mattress. I have never found a bed more comfortable. All those who have experienced it have confirmed its comfort. Friends and family share my view, and some have even attempted to get one. But their attempts have been fruitless, because the company I purchased it from, no longer makes them.

The series of events culminating in my agitation and inability to sleep, led to a feeling of unbearable discomfort. So a little later on, when I felt that I had finally taken enough, I decided that I wanted to go home. I was not receiving any treatment in hospital that could not be made available at home.

I gingerly slid over the side of the bed, putting my weight on my good side, and leaning on the bed table, I moved sufficiently away from the bed to get a clear view of the staff station. I need not have worried. There was a nurse there that I had not seen before. I managed to slowly propel my table across the floor to the nurse's station that was three to four yards away. There I asked the nurse to phone a taxi for me. She promised to dial the number; I waited a short while by the desk, while she appeared to dial the number. I continued to wait for a couple of minutes. She turned to me and said that there was no one there.

I thought her response was strange, because the taxi office was always staffed, 24 hours a day. It was a 24 hour service, and the phone was always attended. I did not believe a nurse would lie. Perhaps the receptionist or another person on duty at the taxi office had gone out temporarily, possibly to the toilet. I asked the nurse to try again in a few minutes time, and shared that I would call back later.

Over five minutes later, I started out to get back to the nurses station. It was easier this time, because I had the use of a zimmer frame. The Asian patient neighbour to my left, who used to wander, had left a frame next to my bed. Although it was lighter and more manoeuvrable than my table, it meant a longer journey, which meant going around the bed rather than straight to the nurse's station which was right in front of my bed.

About half way to the nurses' station, the gladiator looking one, appeared from the left, and dragged the zimmer frame out of my hands. I was horrified. It was unexpected - totally out of the blue. We both looked directly at each other and I saw her eyes grow wide with surprise. An initial wave of confusion flowed through me, until I saw her look me up and down. Then a cold understanding dawned on me. With my support removed I was meant to fall, and to suffer in my paralyses.

My vulnerability was being used against me. If I had fallen, my helplessness would have been graphically highlighted as I attempted, unsuccessfully, to stand. I was meant to be blown away by humiliation. So she was terribly surprised when I did not fall. Despite her removing my support, I had remained standing. I could not understand it myself. But it was not over yet. I had turned to the left when I was been dealt with by the gladiator looking nurse. As I returned my attention to getting back to my bed, I felt a blow to my stomach.

I looked up, and was shocked to see the nurse who I thought was in charge, the "sister". She had chucked me. A chuck is a double handed punch, favoured by Jamaicans. It can either be a heavy push, and a prelude to serious violence or it can be the commencement of the thing itself.

I did not know which one my Chuck was, but it was forceful enough to register pain. I was speechless, I could not believe it. I had never thought such a thing possible. Nothing had prepared me for this. My impressions of hospital were based on a childhood experience of having my tonsils removed. It was a place you went, to be looked after by smiling people and where you got a chance to eat lots of ice cream for afters.

Now my sense of the real was shaken to its foundations, and suspended as if trapped in another universe in another dimension. Overwhelmed, all thoughts left me. I did not know what to do, and even if I had known, my volition had evaporated. Time stood still. My paralysis had left me unable to defend myself physically. But it would never have crossed my mind to retaliate, and to attack a member of the medical staff. Furthermore, they were all women; I couldn't retaliate against women.

Anyway, my condition was such that I was still too weak to fight. But, if this was a war, however weird it felt, I had achieved a victory. I was still on my feet, still standing. They had assaulted me, but had failed to humiliate me as they had intended. That must have given them something to think about. I have no logical explanation for my remaining standing. I should by all accounts have gone down from one or other of the two assaults. It remains the great mystery of my life, and I shall thank the almighty all of my days.

What was I going to do? I must have done something wrong. I must be to blame in some way. But I was too ashamed to contemplate speaking to or telling anyone about my experience. I had to get away from exposure to this type of treatment immediately. But I would need to get help from outside the ward and hospital. It was a matter of safety. Even by crawling, apart from the humiliation, it would not be possible for me to reach the ward entrance door. I could not get away from the ward.

Yes! It had to be the bed for the present, I had little choice. Even so I had not encountered any violence while in bed. I would be safe there, providing I did not take any medication, food or drink from the late night staff. But how was I going to get to the bed without support, something to lean onto. I found unexpectedly that I had more strength in both legs, than I had previously thought. By swinging my hips, I could lift and reach forward with my good left leg, drag my mostly paralyzed right leg forwards, rebalance and then repeat the manoeuvre.

Using this rather unorthodox style of locomotion, I managed to make my way back towards the bed. Fortunately it was only a short distance away. Almost there, I lunged forward to crash on top of the bed in exhaustion. Luckily the cot sides were down. That night I thought endlessly, about what I could possibly have done wrong. I could think of nothing, I had complied with everything requested of me, without any protest. I had always been polite.

I could find no reason for their behaviour. It was like a science fiction programme on TV, "Doctor Who", which used to scare me as a child. It was one of two things on television that was guaranteed to give me night-mares. The other was "The Outer Limits" (1963), which used to introduce itself, by asking you not to adjust your set, and informing you, that they had control. This was a precursor to repeated presentation of the bizarre as real, and suggesting like Shakespeare's, in "Hamlet", that there existed more in reality, than in our imagination. It was like, being part of a nightmare tale, by Edgar Allen Poe, the 19th century horror writer, (1807-1849) who specialised in tales of the supernatural. It was not real. I would re-enter my dream and when I woke up the following day, it would all be gone.

Inappropriate behaviour by me did not appear on the cards. Otherwise, it would have been brought to my attention in some specific verbal way; or was this simply the NHS, in the 21st Century. Had I been away from hospitals, for so long, I had been unaware of the changes that had taken place. But that could not be the case either; otherwise there would be a huge scandal, and, with political repercussions; which I along with other members of the general public, would certainly learn about. I was avid about the 6.00pm news on, BBC 1, and the 7.00pm on Channel 4. I would have heard.

Years ago I had heard rumours mentioned on TV, and in the press, of vulnerable patients being mistreated in NHS hospitals. But these were confined to geriatric and mental health patients, as they were referred to at the time. But I had not heard such stories, about general wards, and this ward was a general one. Anyway, whatever was behind the treatment I had received, it was abuse, and I was not going to take more. But what was I going to do to avoid it.

The following day I came to life at 5.00am and finished off my water in a transparent, blue plastic jug. I noticed that it was collected by a ward helper each day, just after eight am. It was not returned until well into the morning. If you hadn't drunk your fill before it was removed, you could suffer. I then surveyed the assortments on my table, and ate some biscuits and several fruit, excluding apples, because my remaining teeth could not manage them, without being at risk. In this way I tried to hurry the day along.

After I had eaten and drunk; I tried to go back to sleep but to no avail. So I tried to remain mute, until a kinder hour. At a little after 8.00am, the tomboyish, white staff nurse, approached my bed, and signalled that it was time for a wash. She had brought a wheel chair, and she helped me into it. She wheeled me into the bathroom, which had both toilet and shower. We turned left inside the bathroom to the shower.

I had no reasons to feel wary, because I had experienced ill treatment only at the hands of late night, Jamaican Black staff. In any case my normal attitude to medical staff is to respect, trust, and cooperate. She gave me a length of blue and white nylon and cotton composite, designed to look like a cloth, to wash my front, using my better hand. She helped with the parts I could not reach. It was so relaxing not to have to be on your guard.

It was on the way back that I noticed it: A big red and black hazard sign. It was stuck about four feet up my curtains, for all to behold, on either side of that section of the ward. In social work, in which I had been involved, for many years, we were used to using hazard warnings. They meant that the person who it applied to, was likely to cause trouble, or was dangerous and could harm. I was none of those. Who had put it up, and why? It was not like the yellow or orange ones which were used to warn of wet and slippery surfaces. I rationalized that although the colour was different it meant the same. I was not going to make a fuss. People would be able to form their own opinion, for themselves, as to what I was like. They would make their own judgments. However despite my reason, I could not help feeling flickers, of puzzlement and anxiety. What was going on? How far did it stretch?

THE BREAKFAST PEOPLE

The experience of the late night staff had left me too traumatised to want to have much to do with anyone who looked as if they belonged to that crew. I preferred to avoid them, even if it was an offer of assistance. Consequently, I decided to make my own way to the bathroom and shower, unaided by anyone. I would set out just after 7.00pm each day, soon after they had gone. I did not have far to go. The bath room was just behind the nurses' station. I clung on to things most of the way; for the remainder, I found that my paralysed leg was getting stronger and I could half drag it the few feet of open ward, where nothing was available to hang on to.

After my shower, I either went to the day room or returned to my bed, and laid on top. I could never get comfortable in the imitation leather, plastic chairs. These appeared to come in three colours, but mostly greyish green. They were allocated one to each bed except the day room, where they provided generous seating for groups. Their colour and lack of comfort, was an ongoing reminder of an institutional setting.

Most days however, I would make myself scarce from the open ward, by going to the day room immediately after my morning shower. I would stay there most of the day, almost every day. Even my hospital meals were brought to me there. Breakfast came early in the day. The domestic staff consisted of four people who took turns to serve it. They rotated every few days, when members of the group were called to other duties.

The one who came most often was a handsome, chiselled face, white woman, of above average height. She was quiet, until one morning I noticed that she had a tattoo on one arm. I commented about it and she told me she liked tattoos. I spontaneously asked her if she had any more. She pulled a sleeve up her shirt to show me another one high up on her shoulder, drifting towards her back.

Despite there being only the two of us in the room, I was surprised how readily she did this. She must have been very proud of them. I decided I had better not ask her if she had any more. Perhaps the two she showed me were the only ones she had, and she was so proud of them, she wanted to show them off. I had no way of knowing, but I was not going to risk being accused of acting inappositely with NHS staff.

When she disappeared for longer than usual I found myself looking around for her. Then suddenly, out of the blue, one lunch time, she appeared and brought me an apple. It was one of the green and crunchy varieties. It was sweet enough, but I had to treat it with respect because of my fragile front teeth. After that I began to think of her as a near friend. However, several days afterwards when I saw her in the corridor opposite the ward entrance, it was natural for me to say hello.

But she ignored me. Her reaction reminded me of white friends at school, who once they were out of the gates, would walk on the other side of the road if they saw you approaching. So I should not have been surprised, but I was. I thought this sort of attitude had disappeared a long time ago. Obviously I was wrong.

The only male among the staff, who served me breakfast, and sometimes dinner, was a young white man. He was a large person who invariably dressed in blue and looked very sad, until you showed an interest in him. But he wore such a defensive aura that it took an effort to approach him. On a particularly nasty day where it rained continuously, I managed to engage him in conversation about the weather. I realised that he was actually a shy, gentle, person. From there on we would nod to or greet each other, whenever we met, regardless of the task he was engaged with or the setting. No one else appeared to speak to him and I sensed that he was very lonely.

There was also a little Asian woman among the regulars of the breakfast group. She was outgoing and often initiated the conversation, and would ask where you had been if she had not seen you for a few days. However, most of her sentences were shaped as questions. This tended to limit conversations to a yes or no response. She was trying so hard to fulfil her role and to do the right thing, that you could not help overlooking her verbal shortcomings.

Sometimes a pretty, plump, teenage girl was part of the breakfast crew. She would come for a few days and then you would not see her again for weeks. When she came she would pay so much attention to the scales, which were normally kept in the room, so that I eventually made a point of telling her that, she was OK.

I liked the breakfast crew because apart from a few of the medical staff, they were easy to relate to. You could relax and converse with them, at a normal human level without medic labels, acting as a barrier to ordinary human contact.

This had been noted by "Shaz", the social psychologist, a long time ago. He had undertaken research into the relationship between patients and staff in mental health and allied institutions. He had found similarly, that patients related better to non-professional staff. There was also another reason why I liked the breakfast people, as well as finding them easy to relate to. They were one of the few people who varied the list, so that I regularly got served almost first, instead of the other way around, at both breakfast and dinner times.

The Physiotherapists

I was rescued periodically by the physiotherapists or physios, as everyone used to call them. They took me away from the ongoing tedium and sameness, laced with anxiety, about the late night staff. They would collect me several times a week and wheel me up the ward to their unit. They did this for the first half of my stay in hospital, until I became mobile sufficiently to make my own way to their base. They were usually in twos. The pair who used to collect me were both athletic built and were a white female and a fit looking, young white man. This pair escorted me to the unit on my first visit. Inside the unit was another male physio, who was patiently, helping a male patient to stand, with the support of double rails.

Sitting and writing at a desk, on the right hand side as you came through the front door of the unit, was a pretty Black nurse, who when I later spoke to her, turned out to be Jamaican. As she stood up, I could see that she had well defined legs that were rather nice. This was perhaps another benefit of their athleticism. All four were above average height and looked as if they took their business seriously. They undoubtedly practiced their arts, not only on the patients, but on themselves as well.

They soon had me doing a range of ingenious exercises, which commenced with my moving the toes and heel of my bad foot into different positions. I had faith in them, but I must confess I was a bit sceptical of these exercises at first. Surprisingly they definitely helped, because, after a few sessions of their contortions, my bad leg became more mobile. My rate of progress surprised even them. I had faith in prayer, and I was not surprised at my remarkably fast improvement, because I was a Pentecostal Christian. We believe in the power of prayer, and I knew that many people, including family, friends, the neighbours from my cul-de-sac, plus the congregation of at least two churches, were all praying for me. I was hoping for a quick and complete recovery.

The respectful, gentle, caring approach of the physios, reflected the professionalism and humanity I had come to admire and expect, from the NHS.

THE DAY ROOM

My trip to the physiotherapy unit was also rewarding in another way. It led me to become aware of the day room, otherwise known as the TV room. This I made use of later in the day, after I had been returned to bed, by the physiotherapists. Approaching lunch time, I wanted to be alone. Precariously pushing on my table, I made my way to the day room, which, I had discovered earlier in the day, was adjacent to the physiotherapy unit.

I found it empty. As I later discovered that was nearly always the case, with few exceptions, which included staff professional meetings, weekly update sessions, or for medical appointments with patients. The only other users were the few patients, who like me, had discovered and visited it, when they needed personal space.

When my sisters came early to meet my consultant, they met me in the day room. We spent a little time there and together we walked down to my bed. They wanted a clearer understanding of my condition; really to see if there was some crumb they could find for comfort, any scrap, to ease their concern for me. Together we walked down to my bed, with them supporting me heavily on both sides. We eventually saw the consultant when it was my turn. That seemed to drag on for a long time.

When he eventually arrived, he showed me copies of the scan of my brain. Three dark marks, curved with the shape of my head. He did not have to say much for me to understand that they represented the bleeds responsible for my strokes. In the face of this sort of technology, there was no faking it. He spoke to my sisters in a quiet voice. I could not hear his comments, because I had partial hearing from early childhood, as the result of mumps.

My miniature hearing aid that I relied on, which had cost me a small fortune, had been lost in my transfer, from one place to another in hospital. I then discovered that not only was I without my normal bionics, my spare was not working, despite three valiant efforts of the psychologist and day sister, who kept sending it across repeatedly, to the hospital hearing centre.

I had purchased a private hearing aid, not only to satisfy my vanity, it was so small that it was almost invisible, but also for performance reasons. Earlier I had worn a national health aid, for many years, after I had been told about them by a portly colleague, who was also a drinking partner. In those days a lot of information sharing and social work got done in the pub, at both lunch times and in the evenings.

I stayed public until they decided to change them

from in the ear, to behind the ear. For me that was a disaster. I found the overall performance poor, which was not helped by the position of the microphone, behind the ear, rather than in the ear pointing to the front, as nature intended. The days moved slowly. I was getting a bit stronger, more confident and would push my table to the day room, to watch TV, usually uninterrupted. With my left ear, the good one, pressed close to the set and the volume turned up loud. That's where I met Teneshia.

On that day I stayed in the day room until visitors, including my sisters, came and waited. I can't say how much it applied to other families, but one of the reasons they came to the day room was because they did not want to make an open show of their affection on the ward. Even in the day room I still found it embarrassing. However any form of protest would have provoked such a hullabaloo as to prove counterproductive. So I adopted a strategy of resigned acceptance.

Visiting time over, I was left feeling a sense of temporary abandonment. Not having anything better to do, I lay on my bed and attempted to sleep, but sleep did not come. I had some slight hesitation towards taking my early evening medication, because it involved an injection to the stomach. This was a form of anti-coagulant, the importance of which I recognized. One of my nurse friends had shared with me, that one of the most common causes of death in hospital was thrombosis. A blood clot in my position could be fatal.

I am a coward when it comes to injections; with the exception of the anti-flu virus which ordinarily did not hurt. Nor did receiving sedation, to put me to sleep at the dentist, rather than having anaesthetic directly to the mouth. I decided that as it was not the late night crew I would still be OK. But I was still careful to watch the nurse tear open the plastic sleeve containing the needle.

The evening passed smoothly until the late drinks were wheeled in. As far as I could see, there was to be no disappearing of that night staff, for the late evening staff as they had done previously. But there was something else to seriously alarm me. As the day shift changed I saw the night staff consisted of the same workers as the night before.

The late night, hot drinks came after 10.00pm as expected. The athletic built nurse joined the end of the night drinks trolley and asked me what I wanted. I replied that I would like my customary hot chocolate which she duly brought over. She reached forwards, and extended her arm to put it down on my table. As she did so, like Robert De Nero's knife hand in the film "Taxi Driver", a dark brown tablet, the colour of chocolate, fell downwards from her extended sleeve, on to my patients table. She quickly picked it up, and dashed off trying to look as if nothing had happened. I pretended I had not seen anything and said nothing. But I was deeply shaken, and trembled for a while.

On the one hand, there might have been a simple explanation for what I had witnessed. On the other, if this was evidence of an attempt to harm me, I felt I had no choice but to take responsibility for protecting myself. But what could I do. This was a medical staff whose role was to care for me and that could also leave me vulnerable. There were so many different ways they could harm me. So far, good luck and the grace of God had saved me.

If this were an attempt to harm me, whilst I was on this ward and in the presence of the late night crew, any presenting situation or any treatment delivered by them was potentially dangerous. I had to protect myself in the best way I could. But I also needed to be careful not to alarm them. They were not unintelligent people. Either way I felt in grave danger. I had to start reacting. But before I could do anything, without endangering myself, I would need an understanding of what was happening. I needed to think, but initially, whenever I tried to push my mind, it would not move. My brain felt as if, it was bound in cotton wool and stuck in snow.

Uncomfortable Understanding

The main threads of it came to me slowly. The rivulets are still surfacing. Was this a case of threatened false consciousness, not dissimilar to what, the great existentialist Sartre, referred to in, "Black Skin, White Mask"? In that book he dealt with, Black people, suffering from damaged self-esteem under colonial oppression, seeking deliverance by assuming the persona of white people.

The historical and political locations were different but the dynamic was just as serious, and dangerous. It was mixed with internalized oppression and, intergenerationally transmitted, post slavery cultural attitude and behaviour. This serious, but sublimated malady is common to many if not most, Black people of the Diaspora, mostly Caribbean's and African Americans, who usually refer to it, as a person having "attitude".

Attitude covers a range of behaviours. Some of the simpler displays are, over reaction and misplaced aggression. This sometimes takes the form of an unwillingness to follow the norms of interpersonal etiquette such as politeness in delivering a service. All for fear of appearing servile or weak and to big up or inflate the person's ego. At times this type of behaviour is so contrary to the norms that it lends itself to humour and can be seen repeatedly in many of Lenny Henry's sketches.

Perhaps there was another perspective on the same theme. Could James Baldwin's characters, almost unbelievably, be alive and kicking? James Baldwin was a Black American, 60s writer, who gained international recognition for the quality of his writing and character portrayals, in novels, based on black people struggling with oppression, as in the novel "Go Tell It On The Mountain". Many of these were people, seeking desperately to rise above the pressures of a thoroughly diseased, racist society.

One of the strategies his black characters employed was one of false self-importance. This was a delusional strategy in which, they sometimes adopted the status of their white employers, when they could find work. It was used in such a way as to inflate themselves socially. They would represent themselves grandly, as someone with an interest in hotels, transport or foot wear. In fact they might simply have been the janitor, Pullman porter, or a shoeshine boy. It was a serious business of survival of the soul, under unbearable oppression. Being found out was always a terrible thing.

My treatment by the Jamaican nurses and medical staff reflected an amalgamation of their strategies for boosting threatened fictional esteem and something else, internalized oppression. This was the process by which oppressed people seek to treat other oppressed people in the way they were oppressed, in order to feel better about themself.

The late night staff members were all Jamaican, and either middle aged, or coming up to retirement. In their heyday, when Britain was still a force to be reckoned with; even if they no longer ruled the waves, social status still meant something. Next to being a doctor, lawyer or teacher, nursing was a way of achieving some recognition. So nursing became the first step up the ladder of professional advancement for many of these women. This operated in much the same way, as when the management of the colonies became the haven of the less favoured sons of the English upper classes.

I surmized these women on the late night shift must have experienced the changes that had taken place in society. They must have felt the erosion of their status, and the increasing fragility of their fictional position, but had managed to keep it in a separate place in their mind, and to live in delusion, like James Baldwin's characters. Nursing no longer carried the status it once had. However, they were able to keep their status from the past as long as they were able to live the past in the present. It was more than pretend; it was a type of parallel reality. And this became more real when they came together as people with the same historical and cultural vibrations. However the illusion could only hold together if it was isolated from contemporary alternative reality.

Once I had opened my mouth, revealing an accent and dialect free voice, which many people call posh, I was in trouble. I was the real thing. In their eyes, I represented a new breed of a successful Black people. In status terms they found this a threat. I was Jamaican, yet not like them. I had to be obliterated in order for them to maintain their self-image. My analysis was an elegant one, but it did not cover all the evidence, it was only part of the situation.

Colour, status and accents were not as important now as they were in their heyday and they must have experienced meeting people from different backgrounds, status and accents. They must also be aware of what was happening on the world stage.

The president of the USA was a Black man, and the previous Prime Minister of Britain, was Scottish. This sort of change could also be seen in other important areas of public life, such as broadcasting. Some of the major news broadcasters, on TV, such as the main reader and anchor-man, on the BBC 6 o'clock and 10 o'clock news, spoke in regional accents. But even if this was not so, in their heyday this sort of social change, had been around for a long time. They could not help noticing it.

The Jamaican late night members of staff were not predominantly driven by fear of exposure of their social category, in a changed world. Here it was money, and celebrity status, which shouted the loudest. But

I was surprised when the day staff on the ward, also ill-treated a patient. They were prepared to resort to extreme measures when faced with a difficult control issues.

The Asian man beside me, wandered as much during the day as he did in the evening. So the day staff team strapped him to a wheelchair, and later straight jacketed him to his bed. That must have made an impression on him because he didn't wander around for a while, until he was moved from my dormitory, a few days later. So there was a control issue on the ward. But the late night staff were prepared to ill treat me without objective reason and to use violence. They appeared to have done so with another patient.

I saw the Asian man for the final time, on my way to the toilet late one night. He was on his back on the floor, clothed only in his underwear. He had managed to lift his head and the upper part of his torso, and was struggling, like a fish out of water, attempting to raise himself, with both arms stretched out on either sides of him. His toga was not in place and I thought he had been chucked as I had previously seen them do to him, one night when I should have been asleep, but was not. This time he was unbalanced and sadly, went down. Was this what was meant to have happened to me?

I was left with a sense of outrage at his treatment and shame that I had done nothing to assist him on that occasion. They had done it so quickly that I did not realize what was happening. When it became clear, I did not want to draw attention to myself out of fear of victimisation. God only knows what would have happened if I had tried to intervene. But later that night I went behind his curtains and saw that he was okay. That was also my way of signalling to the nursing staff that I was awake and watching.

When I saw him lying on his back, I immediately moved to help him. I half lifted him, his legs trailing on the floor, to the right, which was my bad side. I managed to struggle the few yards to his bed, and got his feet resting on top, when the athletic built nurse and the Amazon looking woman arrived and took over. I got the impression that they had been watching all the time. I was pleased with myself. Not only had I done a good turn to a fellow human being, I had confirmed that my secret exercise, had paid off.

My fourth night on the going home ward proved to be one of the most painful nights on the ward. Not because of physical abuse, but because of something more subtle. Something more profound! Later that night, when the ward was a translucent dark, with only the subdued, emergency lighting on, I had to respond to a lesser, but pressing call of nature. My better leg had been playing up all day and I decided, to go against my previous resolution, to seek no assistance or to ask for any help, from the late night staff.

But not wanting to disturb others by using the emergency cord, and not knowing which nurse I would get, once again I used my table to move to a position where I could see the staff station. Leaning back into a chair was a nurse I had not seen before. Feeling no threat I decided to struggle the few yards to the staff station to ask for assistance. As I made my way forwards, she got up, came towards me, and met me just before I reached the nurses station.

I asked for help to get to the bathroom, as politely as I could. To my surprise, she just looked me in the eyes and drawing her lips together, she sucked her teeth, as she continued to look into my face disparagingly. For the second time on that ward, everything stopped. I was aware of the vacuum, pressing against the walls of my lungs, and had to remind myself, to breathe. It was almost, emotionally unbearable, torture. Since my father's death, over twenty years previously, I had not felt such pain.

But I was not prepared to beg, or to make a fuss which, I later suspected she wanted. When I had taken a deep breath, I decided that I would not make a further request. I needed to go to the bathroom, so unless I was going to pee on the floor, which never entered my mind, I would have to get to the bathroom urgently. So unaided and in pain, I pushed forward, and hoped that my strength would endure. Each manoeuvre was an act of faith. My strength did not let me down. It held up, there and back. After that I asked for no help.

This was neither from the late night crew nor from any other staff.

Being too self-conscious to ask to use the physiotherapy room, I started using the furniture in the day room, and garden. In the day room I used the plastic chairs and in the garden, the heavy wooden seats, to exercise with, quite openly. It was also a way of passing the time. I continued with my exercises but only in private after I had heard a critical remark from one of the nurses. She suggested that I was "a bit of a show off." I had made no demands on them. They saw me as a threat, and they would not tolerate me. I had evoked serious "attitude."

An all Jamaican crew faced with a Black man who they thought was "uppity," they reverted to Jamaican ways of exercising thier powers. And this also included another ingredient. Violence! The latter explanation for the behaviour of the Jamaican nursing staff, was far bolder and closer. This was right in front of my face all the time. But because of the close proximity, it took me a long time to comprehend the being that the parts composed.

A theme, which underlies in Jamaican culture and tradition, is that of violence. Not all Jamaicans are violent, but violence is a strong theme which runs throughout Jamaican history and is an integral part of Jamaican culture which is evident today. During slavery, Jamaica was the island to which they sent the most difficult and bad slaves, and they would not be suppressed. There were many rebellions and many ran away and transmuted into Maroons. This is a shortened version of 'Cimarron', which according to C L R James, the great Caribbean scholar, was the name of the wild pigs; they were reputed to have loved to eat.

The Maroons repeatedly beat the armies of Britain, to the point where the British were forced to make treaties with them. The slaves kept on rebelling, despite the execution of many of them, and their leaders, such as Tom Sharpe, a renowned anti-slavery leader. Eventually it became too expensive for the British to contend with the cost of continually having to raise armies.

The popular presentation of emancipation in the guise of humanitarian motive has obscured the real dynamics which were at work and its legacy. This is one which includes violence as a strong theme. This has continued within the culture until today. It is admired in popular culture, and is celebrated in music and films, such as Jimmy Cliff's, "The Harder They Come," and as repeatedly represented in Oliver Samuels theatrical performances, to which thousands flock. The assumed virtues of violence is actively extolled as good child rearing, and is glamorously recounted, as in "Diaries of a Black Man." In this play, the most memorable scene is about the many different times, and many different ways, you can have it beaten into you.

This is not viewed with horror and outrage at the abuse it is, although recently there has been some condemnation in literature. But it is generally lauded, for being so essentially a part, of what it is to be Jamaican. Children are not taught to resolve conflict by peaceful means. They are conditioned, from an early age, to use violence to deal with them. They are taught that if their opponent is small they should aim high. When faced with the contrary if they are big, they should aim low, and not to stop until they have drawn blood, or "knocked them out."

This is so universal that, with few exceptions, almost everyone takes pride in speaking about how much their parents, used to "beat it into them." As experience has shown, with abused children, if you have had it beaten into you, it is likely that you will want to beat it into someone else. And many actually try to do that, at the slightest pretext, as my experience in Jamaica confirmed. I accidentally trod on someone's feet, at a party and only narrowly escaped, having it, "beaten into me," with the intervention of a friend. In another incident I was forced to make a rapid exit from a busy street, after brushing someone's side.

When I told my family about my experiences I was horrified when I was told that, it could have been worse than that. I was lucky not to have been shot. Many would even take great pride in displaying their scars or injuries, as if they were badges of honour, in the same way that Robert Shaw showed off his shark

88

bites in the film, "Jaws" (1975).

The attitude to physical prowess is reflected in the way physical sizes, including large people, are viewed. This is partly due to the age old attitudes originated in Africa. Here largeness is symbolic of prosperity, wealth, status and attractiveness. So much so that, mostly women, go to great lengths to get fat. I was amazed to find out, the reason that the enormous size of two Jamaican young women, who had befriended my sisters, who liked to hold court, was that they had taken chicken hormones, which had been designed to fatten and enlarge animals, for commercial reasons.

I was shocked that such an outrageous thing, could be taking place, in the 21st century. But apparently the practice was widespread in Jamaica and among some African peoples, where some women would go to great lengths to get the hormones. And if I was in any doubt, that such an outrageous thing could be happening in this day and age, a few weeks later, I heard a programme on Radio 4, which spoke about the practice and the measures that some African governments were taking to eradicate it, for obvious health reasons.

But in Jamaica being broad beamed is also prized for martial might; as is required in physical contact sports such as boxing or sumo wrestling. People like speaking about their pugilistic exploits, such as "when dem, buss up him mouth, lick out him teet', or knock him down."

Childhood furiousness in fights is viewed as a matter of family honour. Failure to do well, usually provokes a beating at home. Many women pride themselves not only in being big and fat, but in being able to handle themselves in fights against all comers, including men. There are even distinctive Jamaican names for the bigger and more aggressive of them. Some of the most common ones are, "Mammy," and more graphic, "Bull Cow," with its obvious bestial and gender connotations.

The pre-occupation with violence, and the ability to perform it, reflects profound damage to the psyche of Jamaicans and the cultural cohesion and tranquility. This evokes the picture of unresolved trauma of a people who have been abused historically, and who have never confronted the damage from the past, in order to find healing.

The flourishing of Pentecostal Fundamentalism is not surprising; providing the alternative culture of the "saints", shaped for the hereafter, catharsis for the spirit and salvation for the soul. However, the picture would remain incomplete without another part of the composition. These are the attitudes which are associated predominantly with pre modern culture, and also in Jamaica, although it must be said, that similar attitudes have always existed in Western societies as well.

This is the attitude to maladies of the mind, mental illness and learning disabilities. I painfully discovered

90

that those attitudes apply equally to stroke victims as well. The people who are the target of these attitudes are commonly perceived as unpredictable and possibly dangerous and imperfect, with less human rights than other people; hence providing a justification for their ill treatment. There is another element in the behaviour of the Jamaican staff. This is easily overlooked because political correctness has put it beyond most peoples' comfort zone, for serious discussion.

As a small Caribbean island, Jamaica is unique for its achievements in many areas. And it has gained international renown in some of these. The most notable are in, the politics of African liberation, in the arts with Jamaican dystolic music, and in the field of athletics. Jamaicans possess a certain forwardness which, in some is seen as feistiness, but in others, an irrepressible resolve, which is a quality of greatness, depicted in the film, "Cool Running", about the Jamaican Bobsleigh Olympic entry, with a team composed of men, who had never even experienced snow.

The mixture of historical, cultural and combative ingredients is distilled to create the predominant national character. These, few Jamaicans would admit to in public, although they would celebrate it in private. In the same way that they would share a laugh of familiarity, at Lenny Henry's take on "attitude". In my experience, with the notable exception of the saints, most Jamaicans pride themselves, in their ability to deploy, audacious feistiness.

The remainder of that evening of the fourth day, I could hardly sleep. My thoughts about what had taken place earlier kept gliding around my mind like a mental whirlitzer. They may have felt threatened by me, but if that had happened, it must have been of little account. They had obviously been in their profession many years. They must have met and learnt how to relate to people from many different backgrounds. In their actions they were simply acting out their cultural conditioning, towards someone they thought was not worth being treated with humanity and respect, because in their eyes, I was diminished, by virtue of having had a stroke.

This added to the spectrum of factors. But neither the historical, cultural, or emotional factors identified, were complete explanations, for the behaviour of the late night staff, towards me. Undoubtedly they played an overwhelming background part. But for complete understanding, there is a simple explanation. The dynamic that drove the combined background factors, was a social psychological one. I had got caught up in a game of, Jamaican one-upmanship, with this particular group of nurses. The aim of the game was to show who was the "baddest" and to confirm ranking within the group and the ward during their shift.

In this scenario the woman who looked like an Amazon had to attack me. That was her role; to be the enforcer for the group, and to deal with anyone who looked as if they were stepping out of line (the line they had made), and which they were comfortable with. Similarly the sister had to chuck me, to show who was in charge. Her authority depended on it.

In this way she confirmed her position as the boss, the queen. The Amazon and the athletic looking nurse, who were never far from her, were her lieutenants, the other nurses were drones. In this scheme of things, patients were consigned to the role of compliant deficient. They would be dealt with, if like "Oliver Twist," they were experienced as speaking out of turn, regardless of the legitimacy of the request. And if like the Asian man, who wandered, they made any additional demands on them, they were punished.

It was in this respect that I had been a difficulty for them. It was not simply the speaking out which caused "eruption." It was what it represented; a potential disruption of the social order, they were used to. I did not behave according to their expectations, less than my full humanity. I did not act as a deficient. However, having set out my description of the behaviour of the late night staff, I was surprised to find that the pieces came together to make a different clearer picture. This was a typical description of gang culture.

Although I had only been using the word "crew", on occasions, as a loose description of the Jamaican late night staff, I was right all the time. They were a crew, or more accurately a gang. Gang culture existed in the NHS of the 21st century. I had made a shocking discovery! Patients were being bullied and abused by gang members who were nurses, at least on the going home ward, it was happening here it was certain to be happening elsewhere.

I did get to sleep eventually, although it felt as if I had been up all night. I was awake again at 5 am, and watched the sun rise from my bed. At first, faint rays of lemon light changed, to a welcomed, warmer diffusion. This caressed the curtains downwards, as it fanned out across my section of the ward. I went through my fruit and water routine, and, at 7am, dragged myself, painfully to the bathroom. Afterwards, it was back to my bedside cabinet, to stow bathroom paraphernalia, placing the blue bowl, in which I kept all my toiletries, on top.

Afterwards I went to the day room where I watched the BBC early morning news, with my head up against the TV, as usual. The Chinese, male nurse, came up and informed me that I needed to return to my bed, for a blood test. He took me back, in a wheelchair that he had brought. I duly had the test. It was done by two gentle Oriental looking, Asian nurses. One looked like a trainee and watched, while the other did the Dracula, on me. The test was unusually pain free. The one who did it must have been quite pleased with herself, not to mention, the colleague, who smiled with a gentle vicarious pride. Any way it suited me fine, because, as

I have mentioned, I can't stand needles.

I then made my way back up to the day room, where I watched TV with another patient, Tenisha. I ended up staying until after lunch. I had resolved to go home, back to safety, and security, back to normality. I would wait for my sisters, who would be coming at visiting time. This was from 2pm to 4pm. They would take me home with them.

I waited until well after 2.00pm, and watched Tenisha's daughter, and granddaughter arrive, and tended to her. It was a demonstration of powerful feelings, and trans-generational, family bonds. I also watched them and other visitors, come and go. My sisters were not coming. I did not expect other family members, neighbours, or friends. No one was coming. But I had to leave, that minute, at that moment, without delay. I was not exposing myself, to ill-treatment any longer.

Still in my pyjamas and slippers, I decided to leave the ward. I would have to find my own way to my mother's home. My house keys were in my bedside locker and I did not have the energy to go back and get them. Neither did I have the energy to make it either to the hospital entrance unaided. Not even with the help of my table, or a zimmer frame, would I be able to get out of the hospital grounds, back to the community, real life and sanity.

The immediate obstacle was getting off the ward. Fate had been good to me so far. Once off the ward I could see if I could find a friendly taxi driver, despite the fact that all my money, in small change, which had been left on top of my bedside locker had disappeared. If I was lucky enough to find a cooperative taxi, I would have to pay at the other end.

So I made my way from the day room towards the ward entrance. Just before I got to the doors I had to go to the left, where the door controls were; on the wall just above waist height. There were two mechanisms on the wall. A swipe card activated system, used by the staff, and a press button one, used by everyone else, such as visitors. Not, having a card, I went for the button, then the double entrance doors. They did not budge. I tried the same thing, several times, with no success before I realised what the obstacle was.

It suddenly dawned on me. The release control must operate via the staff station. The entrance was monitored by a tiny camera, much like one often used, in Social Services and the benefits office. Someone at the nurse's station was watching me on camera. They had vetoed my release request, and if there was any doubt it was cancelled by what followed next.

To my surprise nearly all of the day staff came trooping down, one by one, and in twos. They all enquired what was wrong, and tried to coax me back down, into the ward. I was a bit touched by their concern, and saddened to have to turn them down. I gave the same answer to them all.

No. This was not to do with them. The care I had received was excellent but I wanted to go home. I tried to explain to one or two of them that things were not well with the late night staff. I gave up trying to explain the situation after I gained the impression that, they were not really listening, or hearing.

The impasses were partially broken by the unexpected arrival of Ula. She had been my friend for over thirty years, and her career had been nursing. She would get me out. I explained how I had been treated by the late night staff, and asked her to help me leave. But she refused. She did not want to know. The best she could do was to suggest that I wait until I saw my sisters, and to ask them. I was shocked, gob smacked. She had never denied any requests for help, before, but she was unwilling to do anything that would appear to challenge the medical staff. It was beyond belief. "Why?" I shouted out aloud.

She did not want to face the consequences if anything went wrong, particularly the reaction of my family. It felt beyond me, I could not understand it. When I recovered from the almost physical blow, I told her to go. I did not want to see her again. I watched her depart; silently and reluctantly, with a sad face and bowed head. So it was back to me. I could not stand very long. So I sat on one of the brown fabric and metal framed chairs that medical staff and the physios used. This was opposite the mini nurse station and kitchen, across the hall from the day room, and a few yards down from the ward entrance. I waited patiently, whilst I recovered my strength, and focused my resolve.

I saw a few staff, use the station fleetingly, and some of them drift off, to the toilets adjacent to the kitchen, further down the ward. While they were sitting at the staff station, a number of them opened the ward doors for other staff and visitors. They did this by using the telephone looking device on the station. Although I could not make out the numerals, I memorized the particular keys. It was not difficult there were only a few keys compared to an ordinary telephone. I even used them to let visitors out, when no nurses were about. Armed with that knowledge, I decided I would use it for myself.

And that's what I set about doing. I initiated the keys that had worked before. They were the right ones. But nothing happened. The doors remained, closed. Vetoed again! I had been allowed to open the door for others, but when it came to myself it was a different story. And this was with the day staff. They must share the same attitude to stroke patients, as the late night staff.

There could be no doubt. I was being held against my will, a prisoner, by the staff. And my longstanding friend, Ula, was colluding with them. I was a free citizen. I had committed no crime. Frustration and anger welled up inside me. Then I saw it; the fire extinguisher, nestling in the corner, knee height, where the ward and front walls met.

The idea hit my mind as if it had flown, straight out of, "One Flew Over The Cuckoos Nest," an old film (made in 1975) about a group of detained mental health patients and who broke out of their secure ward, for a day, after throwing a cistern through a window, to gain their temporary freedom. I would use the fire extinguisher, to smash through, a glass pane in the entrance doors.

So I set out from my position and moved up to it. Lifted it out of its brackets, I carried it the short distance to the doors. There I steadied myself, then swung the extinguisher out and upwards, with the intention, of smashing it through the glass pane, of the lower left, of the entrance doors. But my arms never descended. They were gripped by two strong hands.

My improvised battering ram, never reached its intended target as I was held, from behind. I was stilled momentarily, then turned I was looking up and into, one of the gentlest pair of eyes I had ever seen. They reminded me of the eyes I had seen in a picture of Albert Einstein. His eyes were so unusual that after his death, they were reputed to have been removed and kept floating in liquid chloroform.

The eyes belonged to a tall, middle - aged white man, with a full head of dark hair. He was dressed in a vivid, Lincoln green top, and dark trousers. His top was such an unusually bright colour; it reminded me of, the early Errol Flynn version of "Robin Hood." I had been so consumed with effort and determination I did not see or hear him coming. I was taken completely by surprise! My fragile boat floundered. I simply did not have the physical or emotion strength, to do anything more.

He steered me around and walked me down the corridor, with one arm around my shoulder and holding me slightly, ahead of him. I was so surprised that anger and resolve, retreated like a spent tsunami. The void it left was soon filled by a down-pour of embarrassment that threatened to engulf me. I had failed and in full view of the ward.

We were well on the way back to my bed, when to my delight, my sisters turned up. They took over, and my baby sister, who is the largest of us all, put her left arm around me, and supported me the little way back. She and another sister, Maria, the one next down from me, made a fuss of me, while medical staff looked on warmly, from the staff station, relieved they too had been saved from the potential embarrassment of the situation.

My sisters had brought chicken and rice, biscuits, fruit, bottles of pop and clean pyjamas, as they usually did although they varied the food continually. It took them some time to sort it all out. Eventually, they managed to get it all properly arranged on my small table and drawers.

The fostered domesticity gave me time to think. I decided that, if I were to stay any longer, and avoid harm, I would have to speak to them. They were the people most certain to believe me. They were duty bound to protect me if they could. To me, that was to get me out of there, as fast as possible. It would be a matter of family. Among Jamaicans, as indeed other Caribbean peoples, it is a very serious matter.

Family not only provides the universal sense of belonging, that Wilmot and Young spoke of, and which can be witnessed almost every day of the week, on regular soaps, it is also influenced by historical and social roots. In Jamaica, the inherited African tradition of powerful kinship ties, was strengthened by the necessity for social, support systems, in the absence of a state one, which when it existed, was only of the most rudimentary order. So family members, often referred to by the biblical title of brethren, were relied on for support in everything.

Over time family names acquired the significance of social brands, and the names of remembered family members, would acquire mythic significance with age. Hence, wherever you went on the island, and also among Jamaicans in this country, it would not take long for someone, on hearing your name, to identify your family, where they originated, and to ask you if you knew so and so.

Such is the reverence for family amongst Jamaicans, that

to verbally attack a man's family is to invite a violent physical confrontation, and possibly being chopped up by his machete. And these days equally possibly, a large calibre, American made, bullet.

I nonetheless, felt very awkward and, galled. In fact, it was as if I was putting my manhood on the line. It was a matter of survival. I chose the sister closest to me, Maria, to tell. In terms of family protocols, which meant little to me, I did not want to hurt feelings, she was the appropriate one. I did not want to speak about such a traumatic matter, as my ill treatment, on the ward, where I began to suspect, everything, got shared. So I suggested that we should go up to the day room.

As usual, it was occupied by Teneshia and her family members. We greeted them and enquired, if we could join them, meaning if we could also use the room as I did not mind her hearing my conversation, because Teneshia and I had established a sort of rapport. They were sitting around a table in the middle of the room. We went further up the room, closer to the TV, and drew the familiar green seats at that end, into a semi-circle, and sat down.

Maria faced me, in silence, and I commenced an account of what had happened to me. Her face was initially drawn into concerned contemplation. Then it appeared that she had switched off. Then she pouted her mouth, elevated her chin, and gravely responded to me. She was not going to open the ward doors;

she was not going to help me leave. Time stood still. I could hear the blood roaring in my ears, but failed to understand what it was, until after that moment. My youngest sister, Dania, looked on, big eyed, and nodded, almost imperceptibly, in agreement.

The dam burst. My being heaved, from my stomach, through my chest, and tore out in uncontrollable cries. And I wept loud agonies of tears. I was being kept a prisoner and my sisters were colluding. I could not possibly be experiencing this. It could not be real. Then I began to remember. First the old Victorian accounts of families taking their relatives to be locked up, or calling in doctors who would do it for them. When these were not available they would do it privately themselves. I cannot imagine which was worse, domestic confinement, or the bedlam, of early asylums.

At that time families sometimes request their supposed loved one to be sectioned and detained as being mentally ill. They were able to succeed; with medical and social work agreement, from people who had only the most cursory knowledge of the person and little understanding of their circumstances. Often there was nothing to distinguish between the alleged mad person, and the relative making the request.

What was even worse was that until fairly recent no medical agreement was required for a person to be confined. All that was needed was the signed consent of two family members. Clearly the system had been open to and was regularly abused for ulterior motives. There are accounts of people being locked up for all sorts of reasons. However, my sisters and Ula did not want me to be kept in hospital, for any unjustifiable reason. They wanted me to be kept in hospital because, they thought I needed to be there; for the treatment to enable me to recover from my stroke. They did not stop to think about what I wanted and my rights.

Dania pulled me to her bosom and cuddled me. Partly to comfort me, partly to save Teneshia, her family and any nursing staff who must surely have heard my wails, from serious embarrassment. The physical containment, diluted the acid realisation of my situation, and made the unbearable pain of the moment, manageable. After a few moments, I found the strength to commence rebottling, the stuff of my sanity, which felt in danger of leaking out, with my tears. Then it came to me. It was elegant in its simplicity. I knew how to deal with them.

Violence was being used against me and by Jamaicans. We are well schooled in the language of violence. I would use it against them, allbeit, only the threat of violence. They would not know the difference. I would use their fear against them. They would know that in addition to my family I had other people and that I was, to my surprise and delight, a very popular person: this was probably due more to my family than to me personally. There was hardly a day when

I did not have several visitors. And I even had friends and associates, among the medical staff on that ward, although not in the late night staff team.

The Jamaican community in the town where I lived was a relatively small one. They would know that they would be easily identifiable. My family or I, were certain to know someone who would know them, in the community, once we began to ask around. And as it turned out, even without my commencing to enquire directly, in conversation with a friend, who had close connections with the medical profession, it transpired that she knew the nurse in charge. So I would use my levers to pull their strings.

When I told Dania why I wanted to leave and about the late night staff she was incensed, and she asked me if she could speak to the nurse in charge. Dania was a forceful lady who lived in the United States, having married an American. There everything is super-size and she reflected that, both in her size and attitude. She even gained the attention of the consultant. He thought she was a formidable character.

Dania came onto the ward at 9.30pm, that night, as she had promised. To the great surprise of the late night staff; she not only spoke to the nurse in charge, she threatened her. It did the trick. From that time on, all of the staff, with few exceptions, treated me differently. These were people who had been positively disposed towards me all along. There were two people who continued, as they had always done. These were the Chinese man, and the man who reminded me of Robin Hood. He continued to treat me, with great kindness.

The late night staff suddenly began to behave towards me, as sweet as sugar pie. They even tried to make a show, of attempting to befriend me. I slept soundly that night. The following day the other black staff treated me warily. The white staff stayed out of my way, and looked at me, with a curious half smile.

I was still on my guard against the Jamaican night staff. I pretended to appreciate their advances, but regarded them with suspicion. I took tablets from them, but they were never swallowed, received food from them but never ate unless they were pre-packaged, and took hot and cold drinks from them but never drank. I knew that there was more than one way to skin a cat. I watched them.

It was not just the practical aspect that was valuable, but also the emotional dimension as well; the feeling that someone in a position of authority was prepared to support you in confronting uncharted territory.

He resisted my sister's requests for me to be kept in until my health was much more improved. Their attitude sprang from their concerned that as I lived on my own, I would find it difficult to cope with caring for myself with the level of paralysis I had been left with, by the stroke.

I did not have to explain to him where my sister's wishes were coming from, as I felt compelled to do with the occupational therapist, although I didn't get very far, in my attempt to get understood. This man, although I appreciated his concern, unlike Dr Spellman and the social worker, did not appear to take on board my feelings fully.

So I trusted Dr. Spellman and when he asked for an addition to my numerous blood tests, despite my feelings about needles, I agreed and complied. Throughout my five weeks in hospital he never did anything to make me feel that he would ever do anything to hurt me. Well I was wrong!

I don't know whether he was circumstantially limited in his social perspective, possibly out of a single minded devotion to his medical role, or whether the late night staff had finally got to him, and he felt obliged to support his colleagues. But immediately after my exit from hospital, he sent me an epistle, a copy of which had been forwarded to my GP. This purported to describe my condition, and included a phrase, which I believe was open to negative stereotyping. There was an immediate disturbing consequence, although I did not realise the cause at the time.

From that arrival of the letter the staff at my GP began acting strange towards me. I used to have a warm, human, relationship with them, and sometimes they would grant me favours, like agreeing to ask my doctor for an early prescription. At other times they would make me follow the normal procedure. It usually depended on their circumstances, such as whether my doctor was available, and whether they were busy. I understood and would usually comply, without giving them any hassle.

But from the arrival of the letter, they began acting as if they were frightened of me. Although they have begun returning back to normal, until this day I have to work hard at convincing them that I was still my old self and that they had no reason to be scared of me. They had obviously read the letter and had interpreted it to produce some very alarming and painful attitudes to myself, a few of which I am still experiencing.

In his letter to me, was one very helpful note which I have since used to my benefit. But amongst the other sheets, slipped, within the technical jargon,

110

was a particular phrase that was open to pejorative interpretation. Although I am sure he didn't mean to convey anything negative, in the wrong hands given the prevailing medical perception of a stroke, it could be used very destructively.

Misinterpreted, or in the wrong hands, it could be dangerous stuff. Medical information belonged to medical and other care staff. My notes were not only sent to my GP, but to my occupational therapist, which I also had to convince I was not mentally disturbed by my stroke, although, there was no evidence to lead to that conclusion.

Given the heavy reliance on computer interchange and storage of information, confidentiality can never be guaranteed. Over the past few years information held by public bodies and the state have repeatedly turned up in the public domain; sometimes left on public transport. From my own experience as a social work manager, there is also a more worrying feature. That is the informal sharing which goes on amongst agencies, in particular, the police, social services, and housing.

In circumstances where there may be a need to access information quickly, for instance, to safeguard vulnerable sections of the community or to safeguard the public against a background of prolonged procedures; shortage of administrative resources, informal short cutting, in relation to information sharing, is common, and at times, almost a pre-requisite of getting the job done.

But the most worrying thing is the attitude of a particular group of people who may be able to gain access, most likely through the informal route, to personal records. The police! It has been well known, for many years, that large parts of the police force are racist. The experience of racism within the society has always been the experience of non-white people, reflected in our disproportionate levels of arrests, incarceration, and murder by the police.

The fact of racism has also been confirmed, by numerous reports, including government ones. Perhaps the most famous of these are the Scarman's report and the McPherson report into the death of Stephen Lawrence; who will not rest fully in his grave until all of the truth is universally known. Neither will Michael Powell, who was arrested, without any evidence of physical illness, yet arrived at the police station dead.

And of course there is Jean Charles de Menezes, who a platform full of people saw behaving normally, and people in the tube carriage later bore witness to this fact, yet the police felt able to hold him down, and without any warning pumped seven or more bullets into him. So I did not want anything written about me that would make me more of a target than I already was as a Black man.

One welcomed reassuring factor, was that my GP, who had known me for many years, did not appear in the least bit affected by Dr Spellman's report. If he thought it was nonsense, he was probably too loyal to the NHS, to say it. But his attitude towards me remained constant. He just carried on in his warm, slightly brisk manner.

But my only dissatisfaction with Dr Spellman was when I told him that I wanted to go home, he told me that it was not up to him, but rather the head of Occupational Therapy. I was immediately suspicious because, in my experience, in hospital, the consultant's word was law.

I did not let it stir or upset me. Dania had dealt with the perceived, danger to my satisfaction; some of my stuffing had been blasted to fragments, and I felt I needed time to fix my armour, and recharge my battery, and work out an escape strategy, before I made my move. Dr Spellman's response, only confirmed that I was being held ostensibly, for medical reasons, but in reality my human rights were being violated. I wanted to go home and there was no legal justification for keeping me in.

I also feared that if I did not comply a way would be cooked up, to detain me under the Mental Health Act. He had shared with me the story, fabricated by the late night staff, of my supposed wandering off to the local police station almost a mile away. The tall tale only made me smile. I have never wandered in my life. In my second night on the ward, when the incident was supposed to have occurred, I could only walk a few yards, heavily supported by a zimmer frame or by clinging precariously onto objects, such as my bedside table, for support.

If I could not make it to the ward door or open the entrance doors, as later proved to be the case, how could I have travelled out of the ward, past the six medical staff on the ward, down the several hundred yards of open ground to the hospital entrance, and several hundred yards more along the road in front of the hospital, to the police station. Well there is one possible explanation. But it exists in the realms of fantasy. I must be a secret Peter Pan.

The simple truth is it did not happen. It was impossible. This can be attested by a host of people who saw me in the early days of my condition, and who can bear witness to my immobility. They helped to support me. It was a story made up by the late night staff, to cover their abuse of myself, by suggesting I was confused, in order to attempt to make sure that no one would believe me if I ever complained.

The fact that Dr Spellman appeared to believe them, despite the fact that the allegation, flew in the face of the available and obvious evidence goes to illustrate, the strength of the medical close shop. They were his colleagues, he had to believe them. How easy it would equally have been for the late night staff to make up a story which would present me as insane or dangerous. This story would unquestioningly be believed by other staff and could then be used for sectioning me under The Mental Health Act, resulting in my incarceration.

I am sure the Consultant had tried to help as much as he was able to. If he had understood the broader implications of accepting, without challenge, the account of my supposed nocturnal wandering, he would have found some way to avoid going along with it. But being outside my racial and social context it was not surprising that he reflected the orthodox attitude. The Consultant had simply not been equipped by his experience or medical ethics for an alternative view to that of the staff. As the American Indian says, until you have walked for a day in another person's moccasins, you cannot understand their reality.

Black people and white people have overlapping realities; some of it is the same, but large parts of it are differently shaped by our different experiences. Opera Winfrey, one of the richest women in the world who is also a BLACK American, gave an example of this difference on TV. She described an occasion when she had difficulty gaining staff attention to get served in a store, because they were all too busy following her around, watching every move, expecting her to steal something.

If I get the opportunity I shall try to explain it to Dr. Spellman. But I am almost sure that he will fail to understand, unlike the Asian consultant who appeared to know what I meant immediately. But I will have a go nonetheless. He is a listening man; and he appears not to let his ego get in front of his reason. Even so my hope is a very fragile one. In my experience the power of cultural conditioning, tends to be an overwhelming one.

So when Dr Spellman said I needed to see Hendricks, the head occupational therapist, I realised what was happening, but I decided to play the game not only to make sure I stayed on the right side of safety and that there was something in it for me as well. In my circumstances at the time, but for the behaviour of the late night staff, life was not too bad. It offered care, company, and generally good and mostly regular meals.

HENDRICKS

He used to sit at the work station, and blended in with the other medical staff, nearly all nurses, almost innocuously. Six feet tall, and slim, he had a hale fellow well met smile, and engaging personality, which always appeared genuine.

His name had been mentioned by the social worker I had been assigned, as is customary when rehabilitation is being considered. She was a very pleasant African Caribbean young woman who I had previously met at a course I co-taught at a local university. But I hadn't made the connection, until he came over, introduced himself. He then arranged to see me one morning the following week, in order to observe me wash and dress myself. This was to see whether I could manage safely on my own.

By this time I had reconciled myself to staying as long as it took to show that I was functioning normally. But despite that, I resented the fact that as a free person, who only had the misfortune to have undergone a stroke, I felt I was being treated as someone with mental health issues.

Nonetheless I rationalised that there were rewards in playing the game. Although one patient that I met in the TV room, jokingly asserted that the food was better in prison, and which has been subsequently confirmed by serious research, by and large I liked it. Certain dishes were not only a clear reminder of school dinners, but released old cravings which to this day, sends me shopping for chocolate gateau, and sponge puddings.

Nor was there any need to worry about the other aspects of domesticity. Chores such as cleaning and bed making were all done for me. And there was TV and the grounds to ramble in and meet new people. All in all, it was not a bad life, if one could get used to the endless tedium. The day came, and Hendrick presented himself with his usual friendliness like an old chum. I had been up from early, and was pleased to have something to do. He came with a young Asian lass but she stood well back, and to the side of the shower room, and spared my embarrassment.

I felt comfortable, and went through my usual routine, except with the addition of the use of the bath, which I had used only once before. This almost proved a disaster. I usually used the shower, and almost slipped in the bath. However I managed to recover myself and everything seemed to work out all right. Overall I thought I had made a reasonable job. I was not used to having to prove I could wash and dress myself and did not know what standards were required.

Nonetheless a good assessment was expected. But to my great amazement Hendrick was dissatisfied. I was so shocked that, despite my resolution, not to challenge, I asked for an explanation. His explanation was that he thought I was impetuous. When I pressed him; the only evidence he could identify was that I had cut myself shaving.

I responded that everyone cut themselves shaving at some time. In addition it was not my usual razor, and the blade was slightly faulty. Furthermore that I was unhappy with the word impetuous, which also meant, likely to run amuck; which I certainly was not. I recognised that the stroke had markedly affected my memory and possibly some aspects of my cognitive functioning. However, the word impctuous had potential negative connotations.

But it cut no ice with him; he simply became slightly flustered, and blushed a bit. It was then that I realised that I did not simply have a battle on my hands, but a war. He wanted to see me again, this time making a cup of tea in the kitchen, and furthermore he could only see me in a week's time. I smiled secretly to myself whilst making acquiescing noises. Of course I could use the kitchen and make a hot drink I had been washing and dressing myself unaided for days. In any case, why should I have to prove myself to another person, in order to have my rights, in order to have my freedom to go home!

What twaddle! I felt my esteem, and dignity draining away. But I would not give them the satisfaction, of seeing me vent my feelings. That would be playing into their hands. I did not know how I was going to cope with the interminably long and boring days, but I agreed. I could not hear the TV, without turning up the volume intolerably high. Nor could I see well enough to read a book. The second and third of my three major strokes, had impacted on my vision.

It felt strange how the latter disability worked. It was only after my discharge and during the early stages of my recuperation, that it was properly explained to me, by a wonderful Occupational Therapist. Up to that time I had trouble explaining it myself and almost lost my cool with my GP in an attempt to do so. According to an ordinary eye test, with my optician; my vision was better, and my eyes were functioning more effectively, than my GP's, as he had remarked jokingly.

My particular visual problem was not the inability to see things, but my brain's inability to accurately interpret the information it was receiving. An example of my visual deficiency was that I could actually see the shapes of large letters, but was usually unable to identify the words that the letters composed.

Teneshia

She had a face of pure African beauty and a mouth which spread, surprisingly wide, on the few occasions when she smiled. She had both an inner and outer quietness, which commanded respect. Nurses supplicated to her, as if she was royalty. They would find her and tend to her every need, even when she was away from her bed. I was slightly jealous. I often wandered what her secret was. Most nurses just simply stayed out of my way.

She was one of the few people who like me, would attend the day room, morning, noon and night, ostensibly to watch TV. I visited the day room one morning and was suprised to find her there with her daughter who was tending to her hair. I began to stammer my apology and to withdraw from the room when she told me it was okay and I could come in.

From that morning she repeatedly allowed me to watch the touching scene of her daughter braiding her hair, sometimes adding extensions to it. Occasionally, a small child with two large plaits, her granddaughter, would complete the audience, sitting beside her and watching quietly with round eyes.

Before my moment of truth, and when I realised that my sisters were unwittingly complicit, in my detainment,

I had also witnessed Tenishia in a private moment. She had broken down, and was shedding profuse tears, whilst her family, including her partner, who held her hand, gathered around, and tried their best to comfort her.

I did not normally enter the Day room, when it was obvious that a private event was taking place, inside. However, I stood for a moment, at the glass pane in the entrance door, to take it all in. I never found out what specifically had triggered such an open expression of grief; but her general circumstances, was clear for all to see. She was almost completely paralysed from the waist down and relied on a wheel chair to move around.

Neither did I know whether it was because we both used to spend so much time in the day room, or whether it was because she had also seen me cry in there, but there seemed to have developed an unspoken rapport between us. And then one day, in the late afternoon, quite out of the blue, she told me she loved me. I was initially taken aback and left speechless, although I sensed that some sort of response was expected. I reached out and squeezed her hand, reassuringly.

She had received such a massive blow from her stroke which had smashed her world to such an incompressible degree that she needed contact with someone who had also been thrown into the same maelstrom; to share something familiar and human as a witness to the possibility of making it through. She would draw strength, however tenuous from a dream hope of the possibility of survival, from the most terrible thing that had happened to her in the whole of her life.

She was a Christian and, I reminded her that we were never given more than we could bear; that she would get better and would go home soon. I asked her name and enquired where she was from. It turned out we not only came from the same island in the Caribbean, but also from the same district. On another occasion, I intended to share more but that opportunity never arose.

She stayed away from the day room for the next few days. And I glimpsed her once, in intimate conversation with her partner, as she lay on her bed, in her section. This was a bit further up the ward than mine, and was situated next to the physiotherapy room.

After the weekend, one day, she suddenly disappeared for several weeks. I abandoned looking for her surreptitiously, and went to her section of the ward where I had an acquaintance, from one of the churches I frequented. I looked quite openly at the location where her bed used to be, but to no avail. She was gone.

Three weeks went by before I saw her again.

She came down in her wheelchair to the work station, opposite my bed, seemingly, to make an enquiry.

She then wheeled a little bit further down the hall and looked generally, in my direction. Our eyes did not meet. But she seemed a changed person, in some subtle, almost imperceptible way. Later that day, in the early evening, in the day room, she appeared, more of her usual self.

I was curious as to what had happened to her. She spoke only briefly to say, that she had been seriously ill. Apparently, she had reacted badly to the medication. I took what she said at face value. But I had never before heard of that happening with such dramatic consequences. I was left with a feeling of unanswered questions and unease.

The following day she was gone again. And I have never seen or heard from her since. I have sometimes wondered what happened to her. She had been given a very hard card to play. Sometimes we are removed from the board temporarily for deeper healing and reorientation for a new life.

THE PSYCHOLOGIST

The experience of Hendricks' assessment, left me painfully aware of how vulnerable I was to the medical staff's view of me, through the reality of their medically tinted lens. This was irrespective of however objectively unsubstantiated they were, and in the case of the washing and dressing events, made no sense at all, at least to me. So although I was certain I was able to use the kitchen ok, I was unsure as to the response to expect. I was pleasantly surprised, when Hendricks, told me that it was alright, I had done well.

Having scaled the Occupational Therapy hurdle, I pressed the consultant for his agreement to my return home. He smiled at me and said he had no objection to my going; but to my disappointment, I was told that I needed to see the psychologist first. Alarm bells began to ring. Was this yet another assessment of my mental functioning against criteria that was hidden from me and which would be unchallengeable? But despite this disquiet, I was certain my mental state, which I knew was normal, would give no cause for concern. And I was curious as to what the assessment would be like and what form it would take.

The Psychologist was a warm, friendly person, of about five feet seven, with a girlish face and a generous, pear shaped body. She reminded me of someone from the local university who I had been out with in my younger days. She had approached me at a social work social and was the one who initially made the 'runnings'.

She had entered my life when I had been in the city sufficiently long enough to have buried the biggest and most painful shards of my Yorkshire encounter. And when I was well on the way to feeling settled in what felt like a new environment. I can think of no solid reason as to why she was interested in me. She must have been going through, what the Hamish, a puritan Christian sect in North America, called "the running around" phase.

This was meant as a description of a certain type of adolescent behaviour in some of their boys. However I have found it to apply equally accurately, to the behaviour of some British girls and young women. I willingly went through the test, although many of them were only a little above, what I had seen them give chimpanzees, to see how well they could immitate human behaviour and thought.

I was so bored, and in addition had to contend with not being able to hear or see properly, that I rarely completed any task, and would usually stop at what I thought, was enough to show that I was functioning normally. I managed to keep a straight face however, because I valued the attention and human contact, in the seemingly endless, sea of tedium. And she was a nice person who followed through whatever she promised. She was one of the few people to chase up my hearing aid and express concern about my limited vision.

So I desperately tried, and managed to keep a straight face, throughout her weekly sessions. However my approach misfired, and once again I was surprised by the result of the test. But it was not just the test which had some consequences that I had not foreseen, or prepared for. The test results were said, to be reasonably good, but not the expected ones for someone of my professional background, or education. I had made the mistake of telling them what I did, before the strokes.

Furthermore, she also thought I was impetuous. When I asked for an explanation, she was unable to identify any evidence. Her views were based on Hendrix's opinion. That just confirmed for me, the scope of what I came to see as a medical mafia. Acting initially, on automatic, she tried to defend her position. But she was a reasonable person, who valued a logical mode of operation, and unlike most men, was not influenced by a need to defend her ego.

The psychologist's conclusions had a ripple effect throughout the ward. Staff began looking at me sheepishly, and some, even depreciatingly when they could look in my direction at all. I had obviously been discussed at the staff team meetings and had failed to live up to expectations. It flattened my sails, despite the fact that I had decided to deliberately make myself as inconspicuous as possible. I was beginning to enjoy my curiosity status, and the begrudging attention that went with it.

I had disadvantages in several different ways whilst taking the test. My memory had been seriously blown by the stroke, and I could neither see nor hear well. Objectively it was surprising that I was able to function at all. But I nonetheless felt temporally ashamed, fraudulent, and abandoned, such was the corrosiveness of the dynamics of my new home. Although unconsciously, I had allowed myself to be drawn into the group game, the group could not tolerate none game players.

They needed a way of making you familiar so that they would know how to relate to you. The easiest way to do this was by attaching a familiar description, a label to you. Several roles were available in the game. This included the sick patient, a little mad, the wanderer, and the eccentric. This was usually not a conscious thing. Staff engaged in a process of continuous assessment as part of their professional role, and a part of that is watching to see which description best matches a new person. They are then labelled according to the match.

Staff will then tend to behave towards the patient according to the label. The label has pre-defined characteristics which are known to the group and not only shape the behaviour of the patient but also the group's expectation of him. Because labels are largely pre-determined and unchanging they are unable to accommodate the uniqueness and changeable nature of people. In this way within the group dynamics, both staff and patient are constrained and can suffer.

The Speech & Laanguage Therapist

This was my dark night of the soul, my most desperate moment. Although I never doubted that my faith would see me through, I felt as if I had no strength left, and I could see no sign of blue water. But later that week I experienced three new people, who were to have a major impact on my state of mind. Two of these came in a professional capacity, and the other arrived quite unexpectedly, out of the blue. I had seen the speech and language therapist in the background, by the staff station. But despite her unusual pastel, mauve coloured top, I had not paid her much attention, until she came over to where I was sitting, in the chair by my bed and introduced herself.

My speech had made great strides since my arrival in hospital. Immediately following the stroke, I was barely able to make myself understood. To me, my speech still sounded off. So it was a pleasant surprise to me when she remarked, that it sounded perfectly normal to her, and that if I had not told her that it still had some way to go, she would not have known.

She gave me exercises to improve my pronunciation. Although I could not understand how they could help. I nonetheless practised them every day. It was something to ease the boredom, and they could not do me any harm. And I was surprised when they seemed to help. However, it was her attitude towards me that I valued.

She took the time to talk to me, listened, treated me normally, and she seemed to have an understanding of my situation in relation to the medical staff. I think it was because of her inner maturity, she actually saw me, and treated me as person: not according to her preconceived expectation of a stroke patient.

ANGELS

The situation was like something out of a Laurel and Hardy set. Pal, a nurse, took one look at me, and pronounced, so loudly that even I could hear, "you are a little darling"; and she came up to my bed, threw her arms around my shoulders, and half smothered me, in her ample bosoms. She then proceeded to stroke my almost smooth head, and to tell me that she liked bald men. I was pleasantly dumbfounded, took a deep breath and gulped, whilst I took it all in.

I wondered whether she had been told about me and if she wanted to make a human connection, rather than just simply a professional one. By placing the engagement on that level of humour we could both have fun in safety, and protect our egos at the same time. If things went wrong we could always laugh it off as slapsticks humour. She introduced me to her friend, Sweet Sugar, who momentarily, took my breath away.

Sweet Sugar was five feet six tall, strawberry blond, and voluptuous. Her looks reminded me of the uncut Marilyn Monroe, before she hit the big time. Although she appeared very shy and said nothing, except to introduce herself, she came and sat by me on one occasion soon after we were introduced. That drew a few jealous stares from some of the other men.

Pal also had another friend, an energetic Caribbean nurse of medium height and build, who was also very pretty in a tom boyish way. Although she wasn't introduced to me, she came to my bed one afternoon, and in a muted voice, as if to take me aside like a privileged new member of a special club, she told me in confidence, that what Pal had told me, was true. That she really liked bald headed men.

From then on, whenever I thought of the situation, I could not help myself, swelling with laughter, which at times would effervesced out, forcing me to rush from my bed, to avoid the nurses at the work station thinking I was laughing at them. The ward was full of bald headed men. Pal would be able to have her fill.

My brother in law had been to visit me, before I had met Pal. This made an impression, for he disliked hospitals since the death of his mother, from lung cancer, after a life time of chain smoking. After a few days of knowing Pal, she curiously asked me, how I had come to know him, my response had surprised her.

She then told me how she knew him. He had been her land lord, and amazingly, a few years previously she had lived in one of his properties. So I got to wondering whether she had also seen and met my sister Maria, his wife who would also know her; and whether they had got their heads together, in relation to me. Whatever her motivation, she was a warm bubbly person. She blazed like a sparkler, at a Guy Faulkes bonfire.

134

She really warmed up my flagging, spirit, and so reinvigorated me; I decided to push the boat out a little, and to demand a week end at home and away from the hospital. There was an initial weak resistance, but I pointed out to the sister on duty, that Dr Spellman had no objection, and that I had passed Hendricks' test. This was of no great significance however, because I would not be alone, members of my family would be there to care for me.

Furthermore she must have thought that they could not keep me in if I wanted to go. I regularly used to walk in the grounds which were accessed through the physio room, and which was unattended at lunch times and weekends. All the nursing staff knew about it, but little did they realise that I could not walk too far. Not even far enough to exit the hospital complex.

So she agreed but with caveats. She wanted me to go to my mothers, where there would always be someone present. I had some partial resentment that I, a grown man had to agree to this arrangement, and at this ongoing intrusion into my life. But I agreed, because it was part of a broader strategy for my full discharge without being sectioned.

I was pleased to get out of the hospital and to get home. I received a warm and almost embarrassing welcome from my mother, who had been unable to visit me in hospital, and my sisters. But there were a couple of small surprises. The bedroom at my mother's in which I stayed, turned out to be a lot smaller than I had remembered or expected it to be. Much of the space had been taken up by my sisters' wardrobes and possessions. This made me wonder whether it was viable in relation to my accommodation needs.

There was never any issue about how much my family cared. They had taken great care to provide an empty wardrobe for my exclusive use, provided me with a TV, and were anxious to see to my every need. However, their feeling for space, and their interpretation of my needs, was different from mine. Neither did it occur to them, to find out what I needed.

At one stage I softly asked my mother, if I could use the front room. She pointed out that it was regularly used for prayer meetings. I found her answer a little strange. In six months after my discharge from hospital there had never been a single prayer meeting in that room. My mother did not tell lies, but she was vulnerable to family pressure.

Any way I was happy to be out of hospital, albeit, if only for a few days. So I made no further complaint about my discomfort, and as time went by I got to use the front room during the days and at all occasions except sleeping, and even that was available to me, if I chose to use it. I returned to the hospital ward well before my agreed time. I wanted to show that I could be trusted, and I was still incapable of going anywhere. But being back re-emphasised, the keen edge of the boredom.

The Meeting In The Garden

In the days following my home visit I cast around for something to ease the boredom, which despite Pal, became almost unbearable, at times. The TV room was not a sufficient diversion. So I looked for other distractions and took to doing finger exercises on the computer, mostly used by the physios, and to walking in the grounds. Initially I made sure to tell someone, where I was going, and that I would stay only a few minutes.

At first, getting out, which became a daily ritual, despite the fact that it only lasted a few minutes each day that sufficed. But as the days stretched into weeks, it too began to grate with sameness. I would sit in the same spot and watch the same pattern of leaves follow the same path in their swirl to the ground. Birds would fly from the same boldest, congregate in the same spot, and the same people, would lunch at the same time every day.

I too, became a part of the predictable picture. Even though I knew it was temporary, it began to drive me nuts. That's when I met her. She appeared to emerge from the adjacent unit, much like the one I used to access the grounds. This was through a side entrance which looked like French windows. She sat on the wooden bench opposite me, but came straight over when she saw me, and asked for a light. This I could not give her, because I had painfully, given up smoking, under doctor's orders, some years previously, after my second angina attack; which many believe was actually a heart attack which kept me in hospital, for over a week.

She was gnome size and I never got a clear view of her face, but from what I saw, there did not appear to be a single inch of her which was not covered in lines and wrinkles, which seemed to add luminosity, to rare unblemished part of her skin. Having failed to obtain a light from me she searched her pockets repeatedly, and eventually produced an aluminium looking lighter, which she tried, graspingly, over and over, until she got a light. She then smoked furiously whilst she spoke to me.

She told me tales unsuited to polite retelling. But among the milder ones, was one about Molly Malloy, who sold flowers during the days, and her body at night. I had heard it before on a coach trip to Ireland, on a tour of Dublin; there you can see a bronze statue of her, on the famous people and places city tour and which featured the Guinness factory, prominently. She told me tales of unexpected bawdiness, which I later discovered, were similar to those told by comedians in after dinner entertainment, in hotels and pubs throughout the country.

One such tale was of the old man who she said she had met in the grounds. He was crying, and when she asked him what the matter was, he told her that he was ninety, and had married a wife aged 19 years. She had kept demanding her marital rights, morning, noon, and night. He couldn't remember his way back home. After my second home visit, I shared this joke with Hendricks and he could not help laughing. That's when I was certain that my ordeal was over. For if you can share a joke with a man and make him laugh, you have persuaded him to accept you as you are and have always been. Thanks be to God. Normal!

EPILOGUE

My first days at home were euphoric. It was nice to connect with every one again. My mom was at the top of the list. She had not been well enough to visit me in hospital. She had seen me on weekend visits to the home. However, despite this she made a great fuss of me and my home coming, and hugged me many times. My mother and sisters always asked if I was hungry or when I had last eaten. If either they or my mom were dissatisfied with my response, my mom would insist that I have something to eat or either they or the live in carer would bring it.

As the days went by a pattern began to emerge in the arrangements for my care. This had to take account of the fact that most of my first months at home were spent in bed recuperating. My baby sister Dania brought me breakfast, usually a cup of tea and a bowl of cereal, every morning. She was back again late at night with tea, but this time teamed up with biscuits. She usually had a plentiful supply for when she stayed up late, which was most nights watching TV and was always eating biscuits.

The middle of the day to mid-afternoon was the province of the live in carer. During that slot she would prepare both lunch and dinner. She would bring lunch to my mother and myself, and leave our dinners on top of the microwave in the kitchen. That arrangement worked well enough but was dependant on other people dropping in and offering support at other times of the day. It was this component that proved least reliable, so it was a pleasant unexpected surprise when I heard a soft but clear knock. This was followed by a little African man who steered his head, and then the rest of himself, around my half-open bedroom door and then entered the room. He then announced that he was my carer.

Organising care could sometimes be a lengthy thing, complicated by Local Authority organisational matters. The local authority was in the middle of out sourcing personal care and had sold off many of its homes regardless of the emotional cost and social upheaval to residents. I had been told that the social worker had pulled out all the stops to get me a quick service, but I had allowed it to submerge in the everyday reality that I knew. In that place even straight-forward referrals could, and did take weeks.

The consultant had implied that the social worker had acted in the spirit of, taking care of our own, because I was from the care profession. I was gratified at the thought that, I still had a bit of push within the profession, but hoped that had not disadvantaged another needy person.

Having entered the room the carer enquired what I would like him to do. He could help me dress and undress, make snacks, light meals and help to ensure that I took my medication. The latter was necessitated by the effects of the stroke. It had damaged my memory so that I often forgot to do important things. Furthermore, both my hands were still partly paralysed, resulting in my frequently dropping things most of these mere inconsequential but the things I dropped were items of medication.

The medication included a range of tablets and capsules. Some were so small that once dropped, there was a fair chance it would never be found in my crowded room. The medication was a matter of life and death to me. It included treatment for my high cholesterol, high blood pressure and heart condition.

Over the weeks I had several carers including more Africans. They were always extremely polite, respectful and regarded me as an elder relative. However, one was so poor at time keeping that I never knew whether I was coming or going with him and eventually I complained. There were a number of women, the majority of them being Asian. It was noticed that some of the older women were not entirely comfortable in their role. It was the late evening shift that appeared to get to them most.

Some simply came much earlier than the time set out in the care plan. They would then rush off early. It was when these people who started and finished early, began arriving as early as 5.00pm instead of 8.00pm that I decided I had to protest. I was prepared to compromise but I too had my limits. The time slots they were requested to fill, were the times when there was the least input from my family, and when I was most dependant on carers.

Three months after I started receiving care I began to get written demands for payments towards the costs of care. I was surprised because I had asked and was specifically told that I would not have to pay. Being self-employed with the stroke leaving me unable to work, or to collect rent from my tenants, most of whom took the opportunity to suddenly become non rent payers, my finances were in tatters.

In these circumstances I certainly would not have agreed to anything which would end in my taking on additional financial burdens. So I challenged the bills unceasingly but the bills kept on coming. It reached the point where I was speaking to managers of the private care agencies that provided my care. It did not stop there. I also had to speak to managers in social services. It was always the same response; assessed otherwise. No regard was given to the fact that the care was made a condition of my discharge from hospital and I had not been told that I would have to pay or had been requested to.

Eventually, after six months I stopped the carers from coming. That's when things really became heavy. A week after my decision I received what I thought was a final bill. It was not! The bill was for thousands, this was not only for personal care but also for meals on wheels. There was also a threat of legal action if the bill was not paid. I was shocked but I would not be bullied into paying for something I had not agreed to, or to a service I had not had.

I decided to complain to the highest level of management with responsibility for the provision of personal care, and threatened to go to my local councillor if the matter was not resolved. The senior manager promised to look into the matter and to get back in touch with me. I knew this would take a little time because he would be unlikely to have direct knowledge of my case. He would have to do some research and this would take time.

I waited week after week. He never did come back. But I got what I wanted, the bills had mysteriously stopped. During the second week of my return home as the buzz of my return began to fade and the rhythm of the family home got back to normal, I had a visit from two women. They were from the Community Occupational Team. I had been told by the team in hospital that I would be referred to them following my discharge from hospital. However I was surprised at the speed at which it had taken place, and not having to wait many weeks and months, as I believe had become the norm, particularly following cutbacks. My experience showed that some things still worked well.

Having introduced themselves at the front door I invited them into the dining room and left the door open. I thought this would be less threatening than the front room which had an intimate feel about it. One sat on the settee next to me and the other on a chair opposite me. Both women were of average height and build but wore different personas. The one who sat next to me looked warm and friendly while the other appeared cold and stern. This immediately reminded me of the police and the good cop bad cop interviewing scenario, in which the police would gain information from suspects by one officer adopting a bullying attitude, while the other would act as a friend.

It later turned out that the stern one had once been in the force and was married to a police man. This made me wonder how much of the life story we carried around with us was immediately visible.

They shared that they had received my details from the hospital and they were there to assess how I was coping at home and whether there were any areas in which I needed help. My experiences in the hospital had left me very cautious. The stern face therapist and the use of the word assessment set off alarm bells for me.

At first I challenged them about the nature of their assessment and the reliability of their information. But it soon became clear that they were genuinely there to get me back on my feet as soon as possible. The following few weeks I was visited by the friendly therapist, Lyn. I shared with her my greatest areas of concern. These were my hearing and my vision, which had been affected by the stroke.

My hearing was the most straightforward issue. I simply needed an aid calibrated to my hearing loss and which worked. With her support I got myself a temporary NHS aid until I had the deposit for a private one. My vision was more complicated, I could not understand why I was unable to read ordinary text, and see faces as an integrated whole. This was a confusing situation when according to my Optician my vision was good and according to my GP; my vision was better than his.

I had been unsuccessfully attempting to explain this phenomenon to others for weeks after my stroke. It was Lyn who first understood what I was talking about. She even had a name for it. I was experiencing difficulty in perception. My eye was operating properly and sending information to the brain, but the brain was not interpreting accurately what it was being sent.

It was such a relief to know that someone else understood. She had come across it before with other 'strokers'. I was right after all. I was not going mad. She shared with me a number of techniques for improving my vision. She explained that the stroke had destroyed some of my brain cells. Although these would never regenerate and grow back, there were ways of encouraging others to take on the work of the destroyed ones.

She then set about giving me letters and shape recognition exercises to do. I did these for the weeks she was with me and they were continued by her colleagues who followed her. Lyn never allowed me to forget the importance of getting new glasses. She also gave me invaluable advice on the type which would be most useful. I needed prisms.

Once my optician knew what he was dealing with he pulled out all the stops to deliver the goods. He tested and re tested me to see what type of prisms I needed and I think he may have bent a few rules to ensure that I got them at an affordable price. Sometimes you meet people whose goodness seems to make up for all the badness you have experienced in the world. Lyn and the optician lived in that milieu.

Perhaps it's only when we have travelled through the valley of great adversity that we become aware of them. Although we are capable of, and in most cases create our own hell in this life; the revelation was a gift, an embodiment of hope and I needed that.

The whole of my life had been blown apart, physically, materially, socially and it felt as if I had no future. During those early days and months there were days when I was overwhelmed by the pain of the empty spaces, my old life used to inhabit.

When my will to continue failed, Lyn would not hear any of my defeatist talk. She would call me by name and lift me with the expression, "That's not you." Her encouragement along with the prayers and support of family, particularly my mother, and friends helped me along. Looking back, it felt as if I had been carried at times.

After Thoughts

Seek to reduce your chances of having a stroke by maintaining a healthy lifestyle and a balanced diet.

The main ingredients of good health are common knowledge to most people. They include:

Avoid smoking. This is possibly the most important thing that you can do. If you continue to smoke it will almos certainly kill you either directlythrough form of cancer, or indirectly through some smoke related condition.

Manageable levels of stress. Carrying only the amount of stress you can comfortably manage. If you find yourself making uncharacteristic mistakes, snapping at people, unable to concentrate and sleep, you are probably over stressed. These things usually combine to create a snow-ball effect and things can go downhill very quickly.

Having time for exercise, rest and play. The Chinese also place a great value on laughter and even have laughter sessions.

A diet of low fat, sugar and salt, but which is rich in fibre, fruits and vegetables.

Despite our knowing of what is required, for many

of us it is usually only when significant damage has already been done and we see the Sword of Domiciles hanging over our heads, that we attempt to take matters in hand.

I was living in the fast lane, involved in social work, managing my own business, several voluntary organisations and doing training in different parts of the country when I had my first major stroke. It took a further two serious strokes to persuade me to give up the level of work and stress I was used to carrying. Don't let this happen to you.

Sometimes God will allow calamity to enter into our lives when he can see the abyss further along the path, that we are travelling, and when we may either be too weak or unfocussed to avoid it. He has to force us to slow down to give us a chance to become aware of the danger and to take whatever steps are required to change course.

THE WAY FORWARD IF A STROKE SHOULD TAKE PLACE

Unfortunately, there are some people who can have a stroke regardless of the state of health or their diet and lifestyle. There are different theories as to how this can be. None of these however offers a conclusive explanation for this.

This group appears to be a small minority of people but there is no way of knowing whether you fall into that category, its best to have a number of supports in place, just in case. Most of these should be relevant regardless of the reason for your admission to hospital.

Identify someone you can trust to act as an advocate as part of your everyday living arrangement. In case of hospitalisation that person would be available to speak on your behalf. In my own case, when I was desperate to leave hospital and to go home, I had no one to speak on my behalf, not even family members and friends.

It would be deeply reassuring and sometimes of great practical value if patients had access to independent visitors. This would prevent patients feeling totally at the mercy of the institution whilst in hospital care.

People who have others to speak up for them usually receive better care.

Independent visitors are so important in helping to safeguard children in care that it has for some time been a statutory requirement. Although it is not a legal requirement in the health service, some hospitals have begun to use them. However, in my experience tend to be seen as being of little importance. Everything circulates around the doctors, and without a medical role, people are seen as having little relevance.

But it need not be so. They can play a valuable part of the hospital structure. If independent visitors are properly chosen, trained in the role of advocacy and inducted they can become a valuable means of providing the support and feed-back which many of the medical staff members are usually too busy to give.

The above suggestions should make life easier for the overwhelming majority of patients in hospital, whether they are stroke victims or not. But the particular stereotypes and the expectations which are invariably attached to stroke victims, can lead to problems which could best be resolved by independent means.

Mental health patients in mental health facilities have resorted to mental health tribunals. These are composed of independent professionals including some from mental health background, and local lay people. Tribunals are legal entities and their decisions have the force of law. Mental health patients can ask for their case to be heard when there are disagreements between their points of view and the professionals working with them, usually over matters of release.

Had such an agency existed in relation to 'strokers', it would have been exactly what I needed when I was in hospital and felt I was being held against my will. Looking back there appears to have been times when it felt as if I had been carried and insulated against the bizarre things that were happening around me until I could be set down on safe ground.

Reader's Comments

Everyone knows that it is much harder to turn word into deed, the courage and strength of mind that Danzie Stewart has delivered through his words of deed, is to be congratulated.

Life is mostly froth and bubble,

Two things stand like stone,

Kindness in another's trouble,

Courage in your own.

This book 'The Stroker' portrays the courage of the writer, Danzie Stewart, his own conviction upon which he acts on a daily basis, and has lead to an account of his personal experience of NHS administration. I express my humble admiration for his very own mental strength to write this book, 'The Stroker'.

It is known that literature is the art of writing something that will be read twice: and in my mind the giest of this book stands with this meaning.

"What is this life if full of care,

We have no time to stand and stare?"

Lily Price-AHMED

The Stroker; I didn't know what to expect from this book; other than it related to the author having had a stroke and was recounting his journey.

Having read a quarter of the book, I began to question; was this the national health of the present or the arch ages? What had happened to the National Health? Had the economic climate had a drastic financial impact on the health service?

I continued reading the book; re-reading sentences, paragraphs, pages; putting myself in the shoes of the author; visualising the strength and determination, but also the fear, pain, despair, hunger, trauma, prejudice, the physical abuse he was having to endure. Was this real? It couldn't be real. For the author, it was real.

When I finished reading the book, for me there was an anger that people of my own ethnicity could be so cruel; I also began to feel despondency for those patients who had no visitors on a daily basis.

The final chapter brought back the realisation and importance of being visible; concerns in a manner that shows authority for our loved ones, who rely on the health service to keep and make them well; one day it could be us.

Julia

This book brings to life the personal experiences of someone suffering from a stroke. It is written in a light-hearted manner, taking the reader on an interesting journey of insightful encounters; that causes you to gain a deeper understanding and appreciation of the impact of stroke on the sufferer and those around them.

Novlette Reece

An eloquent, detailed description of what was clearly a terrifying and confusing time which has been compelling for the reader to visualise the raw personal impact of having a stroke. Cleverly using anecdotes of being an African Caribbean man ... hair being coarse like crocus bag and the early in-built importance of personal grooming in childhood gives some insight into life as it was for black people. Danzie's faith is evident throughout, enabling him to come through this horrendous period a sronger, determined man.

Ms Ann Maria Ennis

www.ingramcontent.com/pod-product-compliance
Lightning Source LLC
Chambersburg PA
CBHW060930050726

47592CB00003B/889